SHADOW WORK
Journal for Men

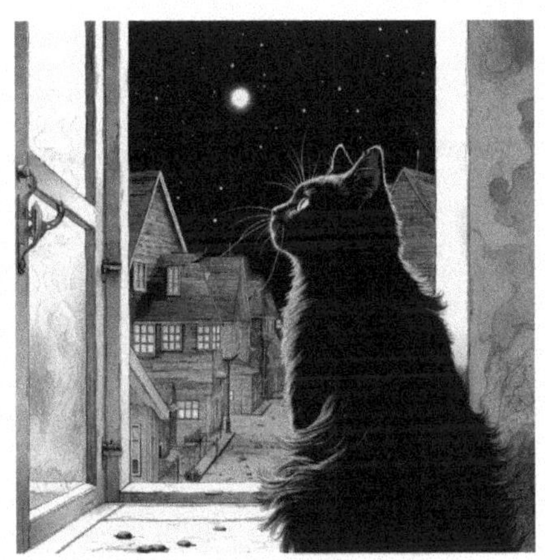

A HEARTFELT THANKS TO YOU!

Through shadow work, you heal not just yourself but also ripple healing to your family, community, and the world beyond.

Writing this book has been a transformative experience for me. I genuinely hope it brings you both joy and insight.

As a new self-published author, your support means everything. Whether you leave a review on Amazon, share a glimpse of the book on social media, or choose to do both, it would make a world of difference. Thank you for being part of my journey!

QR Link to Amazon Review Page

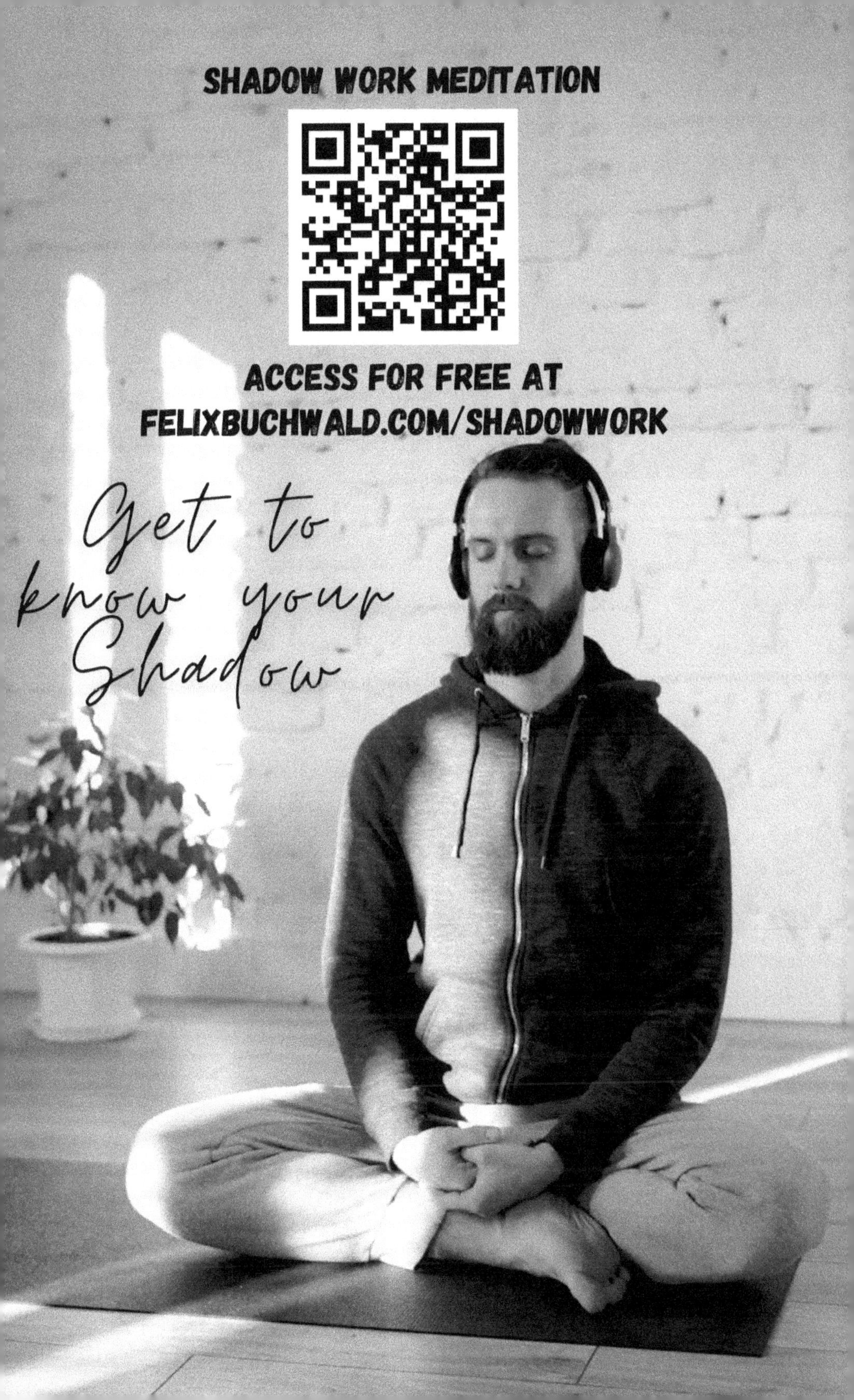

SHADOW WORK MEDITATION

ACCESS FOR FREE AT
FELIXBUCHWALD.COM/SHADOWWORK

Get to know your Shadow

Commitment to My Future Self

Take a moment to sit comfortably. Close your eyes and, in alignment with your highest self, imagine the best version of yourself a year from now. What are you doing? How do you feel? What changes have you made? Breathing deeply, see the strength you've nurtured, the inner peace you've cultivated, and the warmth you radiate.

I, ____, hereby pledge to passionately journey towards my envisioned self. With each word I pen in this journal, I am firmly shaping my path ahead. With an open heart, I commit to each entry, embracing the process with a readiness to learn. As I step into the mirror of self-reflection, I look forward to the personal growth that lies ahead, knowing every thought penned is a step towards that envisioned future. With this intentional commitment, I lay the foundation for my transformation.

____

SIGNATURE

____

DATE

CONTENTS

Introduction

"Knowing yourself is the beginning of all wisdom."
- Aristotle

Gentlemen, embark on an exploration unlike any other, one that voyages not into the world around you, but deep into your uncharted inner realms. This book is an honest, no-nonsense guide dedicated to helping you navigate the complex labyrinth of your psyche. This isn't a trek that promises easy trails or light burdens, but it is one that assures profound, lasting transformation.

You might be pondering, "Why a shadow work guide crafted exclusively for men?" It's simple: along the roadway of life, men are often handed a compass that points towards stoicism, silence and strength. You've been taught to stride forward, unwavering, like an oak against the tempest—proud, mighty, yet solitary in stillness. However, beneath this sturdy exterior lie the intricate layers of your true self, whispering for attention—your doubts, fears, hidden emotions, the 'you' that the world seldom sees. This journey is about tuning in to that whisper and turning it into a dialogue.

Shadow work may sound like we're digging for the bogeyman lurking in dark corners. Yet, it's quite the contrary. Imagine walking into a room filled with scattered puzzle pieces. Each piece is a fragment of your identity, even the ones that seem odd and don't appear to fit anywhere. Our mission is to gather these pieces and patiently construct the puzzle, appreciating the beautiful, disjointed mess that comes together to form 'you.' It's not about banishing the shadows; it's about illuminating them.

This journal is your flashlight. It doesn't just lazily point in a vague direction; it's an interactive, thought-provoking tool designed to engage you every step of the way. No preachy jargon, no unreachable promises—just you, this book and the truth.

Within Part I of this book, you will uncover a plethora of workbook exercises designed to deepen your understanding and apply the insights gained from each preceding chapter. Meanwhile, Part II offers a diverse collection of journaling prompts that stand ready to enhance your journey, regardless of your progress within these pages.

Prepare for moments of discomfort, for they are the precursors of genuine growth. You'll learn not just to confront but to embrace and integrate all aspects of your being, recognizing their necessity in your comprehensive self-portrait. It's not a sprint toward a 'fixed' version of yourself, but a lifelong marathon of continuous, compassionate self-discovery.

Remember, while this book may sit in your hands, the journey is yours to traverse. Each line you read and each prompt you answer serve as a stepping stone towards self-realization. But the pace, the dedication, the transformative energy? That's all you. So, are you ready to illuminate the hidden corridors of your soul, understanding that true strength lies in embracing vulnerability and authenticity?

What is Shadow Work?

"Until you make the unconscious conscious, it will direct your life and you will call it fate." - Carl Jung

Shadow Work refers to the process of exploring your hidden side — the 'shadow' self. This aspect of our identity often houses emotions, desires and impulses that, at some point, we chose to suppress or ignore. Why? Because they caused us discomfort or didn't align with the societal labels we've learned to adhere to.

Originated by the Swiss psychiatrist Carl Jung, the concept of the 'shadow' encompasses all that we have pushed away from our conscious identity. Think of it as the storage room of the mind, where we've stacked various parts of ourselves, often during childhood, to meet the 'acceptable' thresholds established by family, peers and society. These are parts we thought we didn't need or were taught to believe we shouldn't have. But here's a little secret: this space, dusty as it may be, holds the keys to genuine self-understanding and acceptance.

Shadow Work is the brave act of turning the handle of this room, stepping inside and really examining what's there. It's about recognizing, understanding, and embracing these exiled parts of ourselves. It involves asking those tough questions: Why do certain situations trigger disproportionate emotions? What's driving our self-doubt, aggression or fear?

Engaging in Shadow Work isn't about eradicating our shadows; instead, it's about integration and balance. It's acknowledging that we're not one-dimensional but beautifully complex beings with a full spectrum of emotions and traits.

This process allows us to dismantle our old, possibly deceptive, self-narratives and rebuild with authenticity. It's the psychological equivalent of having a heartfelt conversation with a long-estranged friend: it can be awkward, challenging but is ultimately deeply rewarding.

How does one engage in Shadow Work? Primarily, through the powerful practice of journaling, an introspective process that serves as a mirror, reflecting your thoughts, emotions and the hidden recesses of your psyche. While Shadow Work can also be complemented by methods like meditation, artistic expression or therapy, journaling stands out as a deeply personal, direct, and powerful way to dialogue with your inner self. This approach isn't about following a strict set of rules; it's about allowing your authenticity to flow onto the pages, creating a tangible record of your journey into the self. Each person's journaling path is as unique as their fingerprint, tailored by the contours of their experiences, emotions and insights.

"The privilege of a lifetime is to become who you truly are." - Carl Jung

If you've ever embarked on a challenging journey, you know that a nudge of motivation often comes from answering this burning question: "What's in it for me?" Dive into Shadow Work, and you're not just dipping your toes into introspective waters — you're plunging into an ocean of self-discovery. So, let's talk about the treasures you'll uncover in these depths and why this book is the trusty diving gear you didn't know you needed.

Hello, Real You

Shadow Work is like holding up a mirror on a sunny day; you'll see the light, sure, but you'll also notice the shadows. These are integral parts of you, the bits that make you wonderfully complex. By recognizing, accepting and integrating these parts, you'll meet a version of yourself that's more authentic than the person you thought you were. It's about dropping the weights you've been carrying and realizing you've had wings all along.

Emotional Balance, Who?

Ever felt like a walking, talking pendulum, swinging between emotional extremes? Shadow Work smooths out those swings. By understanding the 'why' behind your feelings, you balance the 'how' you react to them. It's kind of like being an emotional tightrope walker who's finally found their pole for balance.

Relationships on Fleek

When you understand yourself, your relationships transform. You become less of a reactor and more of a responder. Imagine understanding your triggers and not letting them be the invisible puppeteer in your interactions. Healthy boundaries, deeper connections and genuine communication? Check, check, and check.

Unlock Creativity

Your shadow isn't just your suppressed fears or angers; it's also your stifled creativity, silenced voice and benched talents. Engaging with your shadow can be like finding a key to a room where your forgotten paintings, unwritten novels and unsung melodies have been waiting for their cue. It's time for their standing ovation.

Master of Resilience

Life throws curveballs and Shadow Work trains you to be an adept catcher. By embracing your vulnerability, you foster resilience. Challenges will still arise, but you'll navigate them with the grace of a seasoned sailor.

This book respects that you're not a blank slate. You're a masterpiece mid-creation and every stroke of insight adds depth, bringing you closer to your magnum opus: the truest version of yourself.

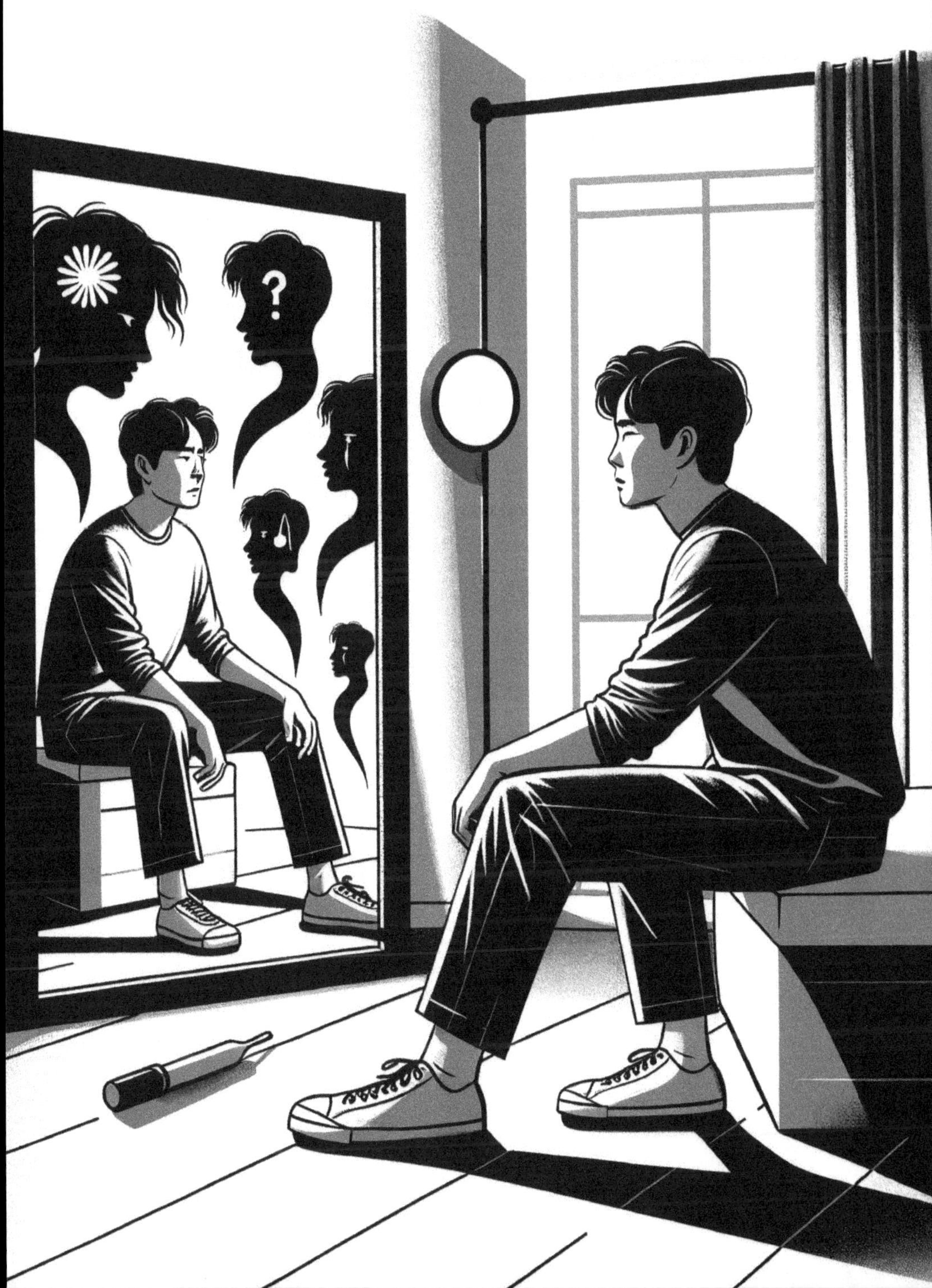

I am who I am and that is enough

PART I

Shadow Work Guide & Workbook for Men

CHAPTER ONE

Embracing Vulnerability: Exploring Masculine Wounds of the Soul

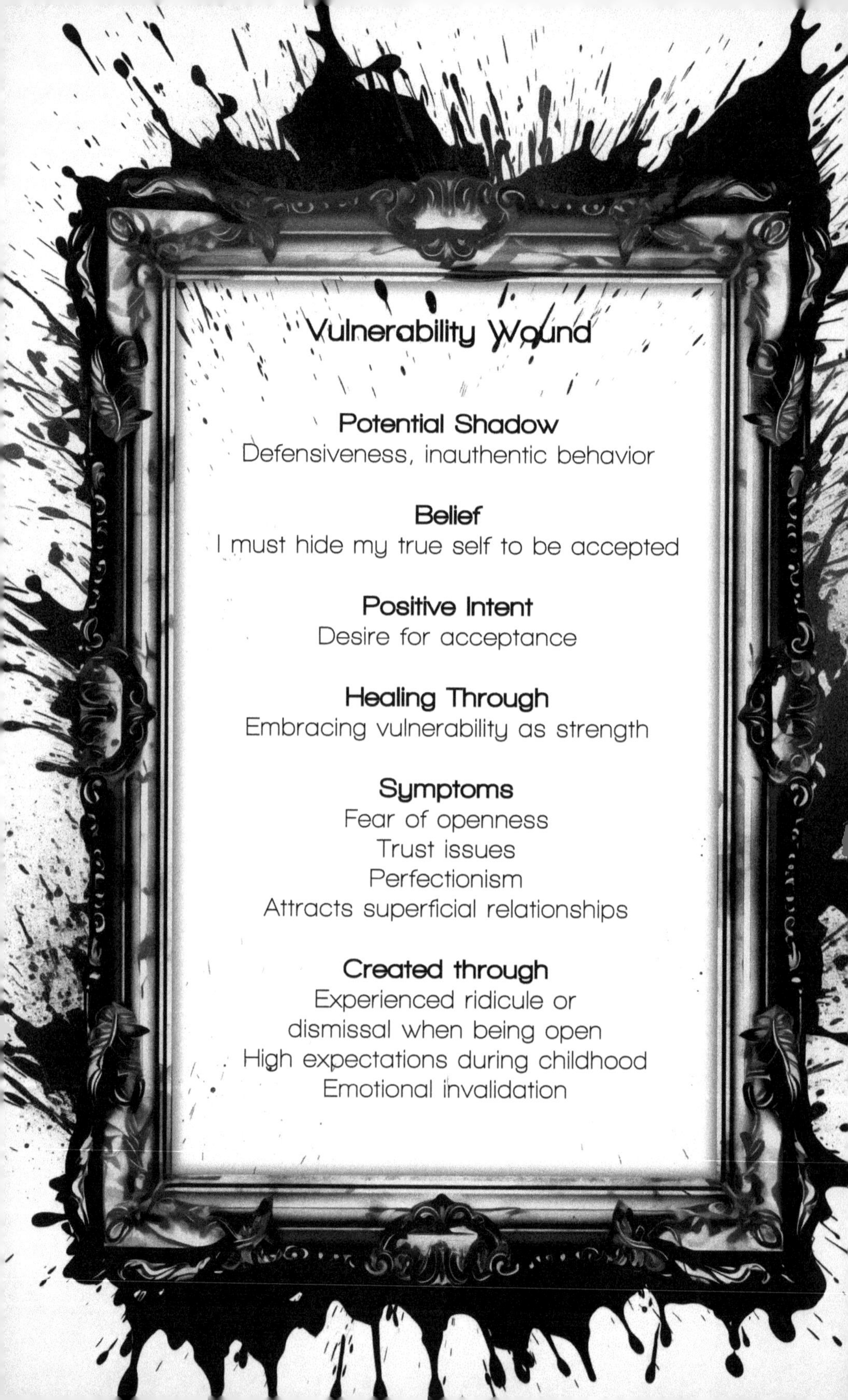

Vulnerability Wound

Potential Shadow
Defensiveness, inauthentic behavior

Belief
I must hide my true self to be accepted

Positive Intent
Desire for acceptance

Healing Through
Embracing vulnerability as strength

Symptoms
Fear of openness
Trust issues
Perfectionism
Attracts superficial relationships

Created through
Experienced ridicule or
dismissal when being open
High expectations during childhood
Emotional invalidation

Vulnerability Wound

"To share your weakness is to make yourself vulnerable; to make yourself vulnerable is to show your strength." - Criss Jami

In the heart of our journey towards self-discovery, there lies a wound that often goes unattended, masked by the bravado of strength: the Vulnerability Wound. It is an unseen bruise on our psyche that subtly dictates our interactions, choices and self-perception. This chapter is dedicated to helping you unravel this wound, understanding its roots and embracing vulnerability as a stepping stone towards lasting change through Shadow Work.

The Vulnerability Wound is born out of societal expectations and personal experiences that teach us that being vulnerable equates to being weak. For many, showing emotions, expressing fear or admitting that we need help feels like a threat to our very essence. This wound keeps us locked in a fortress of our own making, preventing us from forming deep connections and stifling our authentic selves.

To start healing, we must first identify the signs of the Vulnerability Wound. It may manifest as a constant need to prove oneself, an overwhelming fear of rejection or an inability to open up in relationships. Do you find yourself putting on a mask of strength when you're crumbling inside? Do you shy away from asking for help even when you're overwhelmed? These could be signs that the Vulnerability Wound is at play.

By acknowledging the Vulnerability Wound, we start the process of healing. It involves digging deep into past experiences, societal conditioning and internal dialogues that have led to the creation of this wound.

Healing the Vulnerability Wound is not about eradicating vulnerability; rather, it is about embracing it as a strength. By allowing ourselves to be vulnerable, we foster authenticity, empathy and connection. This transformative shift can be achieved through expressing yourself authentically and being open about your feelings with trusted friends, family or a therapist.

As you embark on this transformative journey, remember that healing is not linear. Embracing your vulnerability is an ongoing process, a dance between the shadows and the light. By working through it, you are taking a powerful step towards a more authentic, connected and fulfilling life.

Conquest Wound

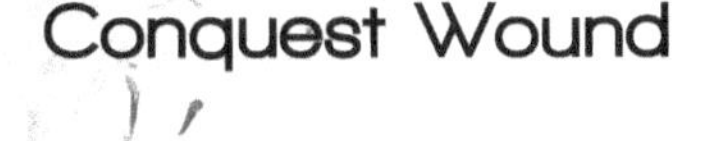

Potential Shadows
Unethical Behavior, Domination, Burnout

Belief
I must succeed at all costs

Positive Intent
Desire for accomplishment and validation

Healing Through
Cultivating empathy and mindful goal-setting

Symptoms
Ruthlessness, disregard for others, burnout
Strained relationships and isolation

Created Through
Experienced conditional love
based on achievement
Highly competitive environments
Lack of emotional support

"Success is not the key to happiness. Happiness is the key to success. If you love what you are doing, you will be successful." - Albert Schweitzer

In the relentless pursuit of success, some individuals find themselves ensnared by the Conquest Wound. This wound manifests as an insatiable hunger to conquer, dominate and achieve, often at the expense of personal well-being and meaningful relationships.

The shadow of this wound is unethical behaviors, domination and even burnout. Driven by the belief that they must conquer and win at all costs, individuals may resort to manipulative tactics, coercing others into alignment with their goals. This belief can stem from a past where love and validation were contingent on achievements, fostering a mindset where the ends justify the means.

Despite the seemingly aggressive exterior, the positive intent behind the Conquest Wound is a deep-seated desire for accomplishment and validation. It is a cry for recognition, albeit through means that may alienate and isolate.

The symptoms of the Conquest Wound are evident in ruthless ambition, a disregard for the feelings and well-being of others and personal burnout from relentless pursuit. Relationships may strain and snap under the pressure of this conquest-driven demeanor, leading to a sense of isolation.

Healing from the Conquest Wound requires a shift in perspective. It involves cultivating empathy and understanding the impact of one's actions on others and oneself. Mindful goal-setting, where achievements are pursued with consideration for ethical implications and emotional well-being, becomes crucial.

Understanding that validation and accomplishment are not zero-sum games is key to healing. Embracing collaborative success and recognizing the value of emotional connections can transform the Conquest Wound into a source of strength. By doing so, individuals can pursue success not as conquerors, but as empathetic achievers who understand the true value of accomplishment.

In addressing the Conquest Wound, we learn that success is sweeter when shared, and that our achievements do not have to come at the expense of others or our own well-being. Through empathy, mindfulness and ethical pursuit, the Conquest Wound can be healed, leading to a fulfilling and balanced life.

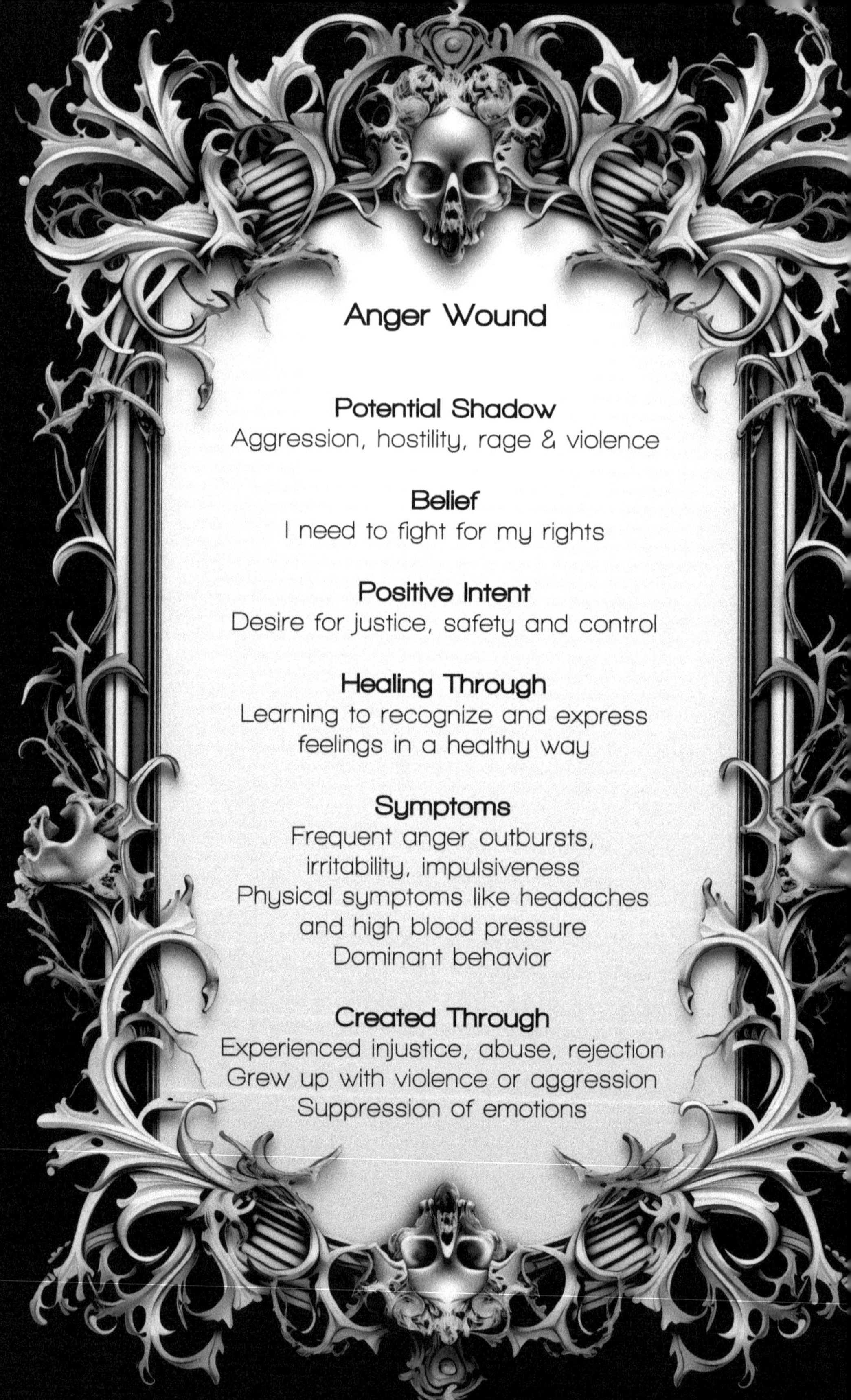

Anger Wound

Potential Shadow
Aggression, hostility, rage & violence

Belief
I need to fight for my rights

Positive Intent
Desire for justice, safety and control

Healing Through
Learning to recognize and express
feelings in a healthy way

Symptoms
Frequent anger outbursts,
irritability, impulsiveness
Physical symptoms like headaches
and high blood pressure
Dominant behavior

Created Through
Experienced injustice, abuse, rejection
Grew up with violence or aggression
Suppression of emotions

"Holding on to anger is like grasping a hot coal with the intent of throwing it at someone else; you are the one who gets burned." - Buddha

In the tempestuous seas of the Anger Wound, individuals find themselves caught in cycles of aggression and hostility. This wound is characterized by a turbulent display of anger, often erupting without warning, leaving a trail of strained relationships and internal turmoil.

The shadow cast by this wound is aggressive and hostile behavior. Driven by the belief that anger is a necessary shield against harm, individuals may resort to outbursts and confrontations as a means of self-protection. This belief often has its roots in environments marked by violence, emotional suppression or feelings of powerlessness.

Yet, beneath the fiery exterior lies a positive intent: a deep-seated desire for justice, safety and control. The anger, though destructive, is an attempt to create a protective barrier against perceived threats.

The symptoms of the Anger Wound are varied, spanning from frequent anger outbursts and irritability to physical symptoms like headaches and elevated blood pressure. Relationships are often strained as loved ones grapple with the individual's aggressive nature.

Healing from the Anger Wound requires a journey inward to understand the triggers and underlying emotions that fuel the anger. It involves learning to express emotions healthily and constructively. Techniques such as mindfulness, emotional regulation and assertive but peaceful communication become invaluable tools on this healing journey.

Addressing the Anger Wound is akin to navigating a storm. By understanding the root causes and learning to channel the energy of anger into positive and constructive avenues, individuals can emerge from the tempest stronger and more resilient.

In healing the Anger Wound, we discover that anger need not be a destructive force, but can be transformed into a catalyst for change and empowerment. Through introspection, emotional literacy and constructive expression, the Anger Wound can be soothed, leading to a life of balance and harmonious relationships.

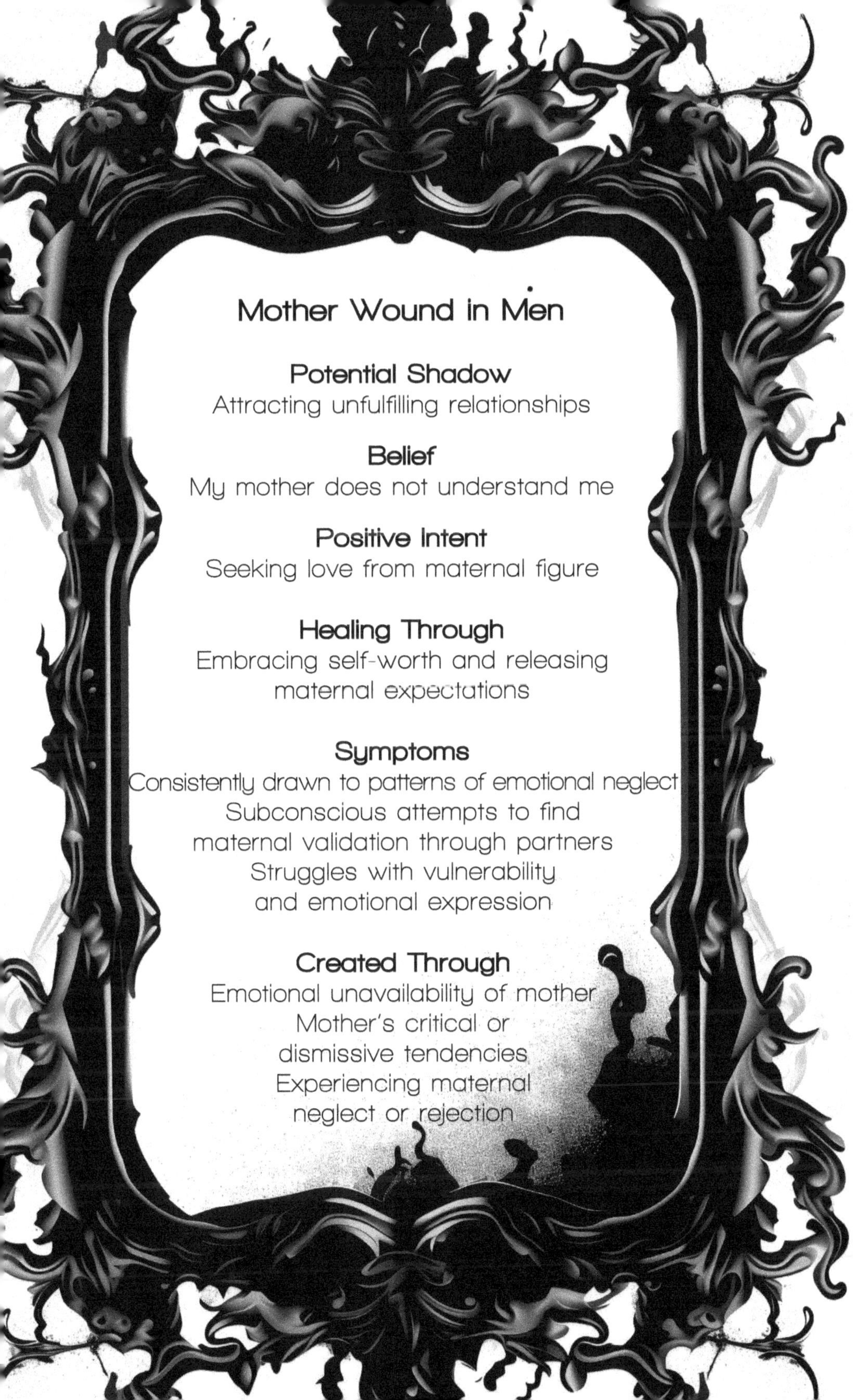

Mother Wound in Men

Potential Shadow
Attracting unfulfilling relationships

Belief
My mother does not understand me

Positive Intent
Seeking love from maternal figure

Healing Through
Embracing self-worth and releasing
maternal expectations

Symptoms
Consistently drawn to patterns of emotional neglect
Subconscious attempts to find
maternal validation through partners
Struggles with vulnerability
and emotional expression

Created Through
Emotional unavailability of mother
Mother's critical or
dismissive tendencies
Experiencing maternal
neglect or rejection

"To love oneself is the beginning of a lifelong romance." – Oscar Wilde

Consider a man's heart as a sensitive barometer, subtly responding to the atmospheric pressures of love, acceptance and belonging. For many men, the maternal bond, or the lack thereof, casts a long shadow, echoing in their relationships and self-perception.

When a mother, an essential figure in a boy's life, is emotionally distant, critical or neglectful, it is akin to a navigational instrument being misaligned. Consequently, some men may find themselves habitually drawn to partners who mirror the emotional void experienced with their mothers. It's as if an internal GPS continuously redirects back to a path laden with familiar emotional neglect.

Building upon the insights from attachment theory, it's evident that our earliest bonds lay the groundwork for future relational dynamics. When a man's relationship with his mother is fraught with misunderstanding or neglect, it might plant the seeds of a damaging belief: that he is undeserving of empathy and connection.

This belief may manifest as an unspoken yearning: the desire to find understanding and validation that was absent in the maternal relationship. This latent hope might lead some men to choose partners who subtly echo the dynamics of their mothers, in a subconscious attempt to heal and find closure.

Have you ever felt an unexplainable attraction to partners who embody feelings of emotional distance? Or found yourself struggling to express vulnerability, fearing it will lead to rejection? These are indicators, echoes of past wounds yearning for acknowledgment and healing.

The path to healing is not predetermined, and one can navigate towards transformation by considering the following steps:

Embrace Self-Worth: Recognize that your worth is intrinsic and not determined by external validation or maternal approval.

Release Expectations: Letting go of the need for maternal validation can pave the way for authentic connections and personal growth.

By acknowledging and reshaping these beliefs, men can liberate themselves from past wounds and forge healthier relationships that offer genuine understanding and partnership.

It's essential to remember that while this chapter has highlighted four significant wounds, the spectrum of personal wounds can be broader. Everyone's shadow carries its unique patterns and pain points. While these insights serve as a foundation, it's crucial to have an open dialogue with your individual shadow and not to minimize its significance just because it may not have been explicitly discussed in this chapter.

Wound Resonance: *As you navigated through the different wounds discussed in this chapter, which one resonated with you the most and why?*

Trigger Search: *In your day-to-day life, are there specific triggers or situations that evoke feelings related to these wounds? How do you usually respond?*

The Healed You: *Envision a life where these wounds are healed. What does that look like for you? How would our daily experiences and interactions change?*

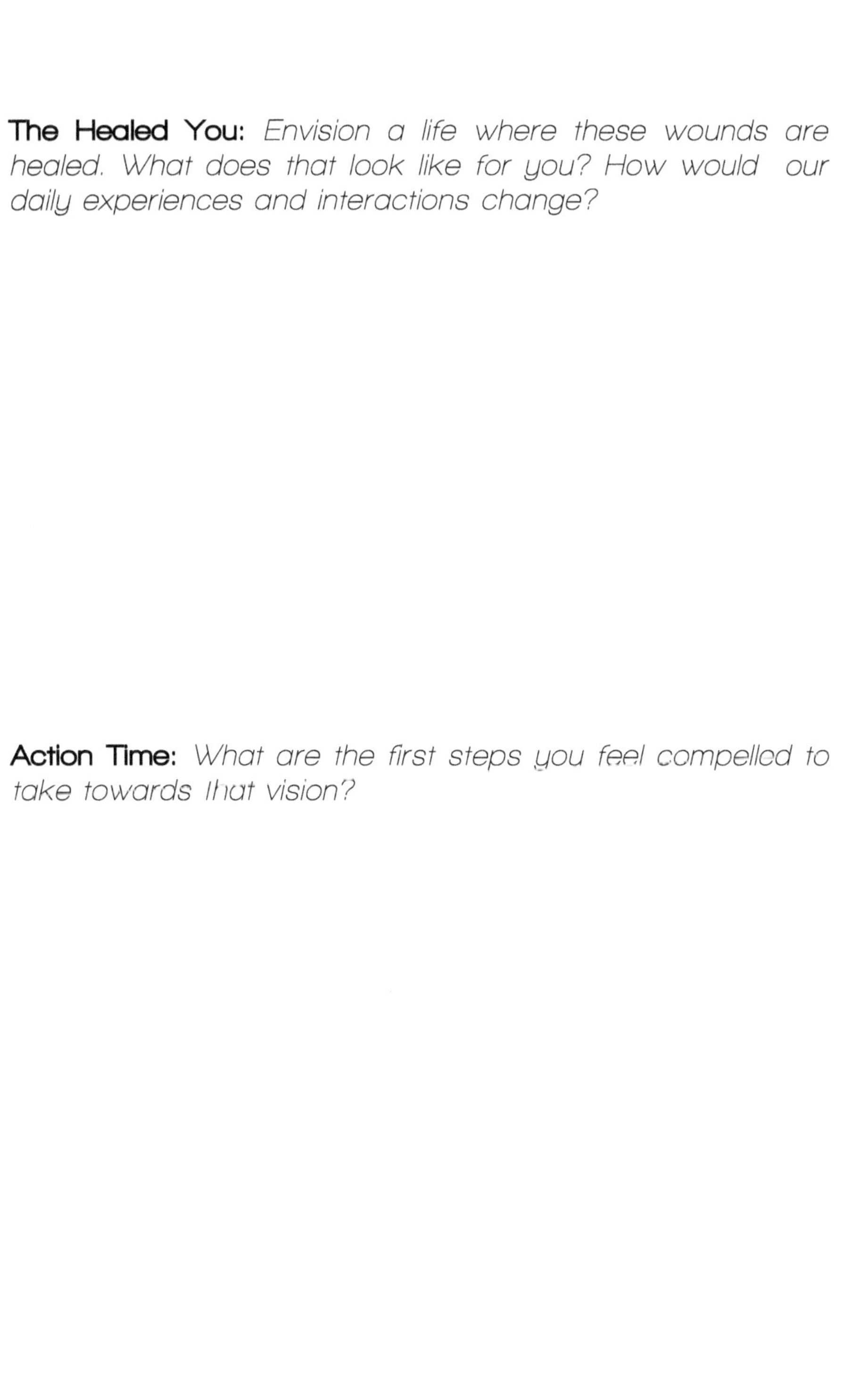

Action Time: *What are the first steps you feel compelled to take towards that vision?*

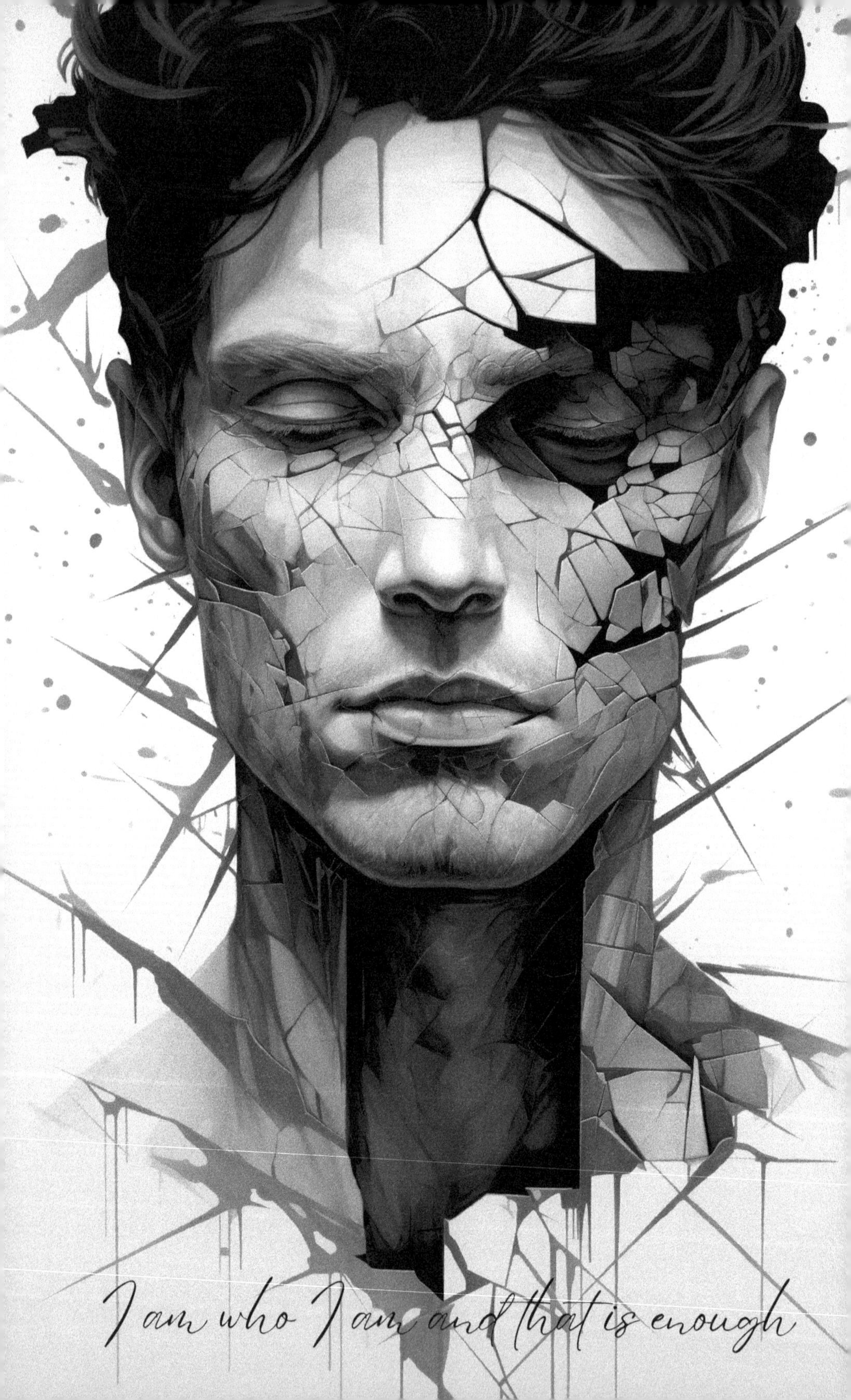
I am who I am and that is enough

CHAPTER TWO

Reclaiming Masculinity: Understanding and Embracing Healthy Male Ideals

The Evolution of Masculine Ideals

"The stronger a man is, the more gentle he can afford to be." - Elbert Hubbard

Over the last decades, the ideals that define masculinity have undergone major transformations. To truly grasp the essence of what healthy masculinity means today, it is imperative to embark on a journey through history, unraveling the layers that have shaped the male archetype.

Centuries ago, masculinity was largely defined by physical prowess, bravery and the ability to provide and protect. Men were expected to be warriors, hunters and leaders, who stoically bore the weight of responsibility. From the chivalrous knights of medieval times to the industrious pioneers of the industrial revolution, the mold of manhood was cast in the crucible of external challenges.

However, as societies evolved, so did the expectations placed upon men. The advent of the 20th century saw seismic shifts in social, political and economic landscapes. Wars, social movements and technological advancements redefined the roles that men were expected to play. The archetype of the 'strong, silent type' began to be questioned and new dialogues emerged around what it meant to be a man.

In recent times, discussions around masculinity have become more nuanced and complex. The concept of toxic masculinity has entered the public consciousness, bringing attention to the detrimental aspects of traditional male ideals. With this term being used inflationarily, it has inadvertently added to the confusion and struggle faced by men. Navigating these expectations has become a challenging endeavor, making it difficult for men to honor and understand their own masculinity.

Amidst the debate of the merits and pitfalls of traditional masculinity, it becomes essential to sift through the noise and seek a balanced perspective that honors the positive aspects of traditional masculinity while also acknowledging the need for growth and evolution. Traditional masculine traits such as strength, leadership and resilience have been pillars of societies for centuries and continue to be virtues that are deeply respected and necessary. These attributes have enabled men to contribute positively to their families and communities and it's important to recognize and celebrate these contributions.

At the same time, the modern age calls for a reevaluation and evolution of certain ideals, incorporating qualities such as empathy, emotional expression and vulnerability. By striking this balance, we can appreciate and honor the enduring aspects of masculinity while also embracing the transformative journey towards a more inclusive and holistic understanding of manhood.

"To be yourself in a world that is constantly trying to make you something else is the greatest accomplishment." - Ralph Waldo Emerson

Embarking on the journey towards healthy masculinity begins with honoring and valuing your own sense of manhood. It's about recognizing the inherent worth and dignity that comes with understanding that your unique expression of manhood is valid and valuable. Embracing the journey means cherishing the positive facets of masculinity, such as strength, courage, will and determination, while simultaneously cultivating qualities like compassion, empathy and kindness.

Valuing your masculinity involves giving yourself permission to explore and define what being a man means to you, free from societal constraints or stereotypes. It means respecting the diversity in masculine expressions and understanding that there is no singular way to be a man. Whether it's through leadership, caregiving, creativity or collaboration, your unique expression of masculinity is something to be celebrated and respected.

In honoring and valuing your masculinity, you set a foundation for growth and transformation. This initial step allows you to approach the journey with a sense of self-respect and empowerment, creating a positive starting point for the exploration and embracing of healthy masculinity. By acknowledging the value in your own masculinity, you pave the way for a journey that is enriching and fulfilling, allowing you to be an authentic and positive force in your own life and in the lives of others.

"The greatest deception men suffer is from their own opinions." - Leonardo da Vinci

In the pursuit of understanding the multifaceted aspects of masculinity, it is important to comprehend the concept of 'toxic masculinity.' This term has gained prominence in recent years, often used to spotlight behaviors and attitudes that are deemed harmful not only to men but also to society at large.

Toxic masculinity refers to a set of cultural norms and expectations around traditional male behavior that, In their extreme, can lead to detriment and dysfunction. It is characterized by an adherence to rigid gender roles, suppression of emotions, dominance over others and a disdain for perceived weakness. This archetype propels the notion that men must always be in control, unemotional and assertive, often at the cost of their own well-being and the well-being of others.

It's important to clarify that the term 'toxic masculinity' does not imply that masculinity in itself is toxic. Instead, it points to certain expressions of masculinity that have been distorted or exaggerated to the point of causing harm. For instance, while confidence and assertiveness can be positive traits, when they morph into arrogance and aggression, they become problematic.

In the realm of Shadow Work, understanding toxic masculinity involves exploring the subconscious to uncover and examine these ingrained beliefs and behaviors. It's about recognizing the ways in which these patterns have been internalized and how they may be influencing one's actions and relationships. By bringing these shadows into the light, individuals can begin the process of healing and transformation.

Addressing toxic masculinity requires a delicate balance of acknowledging the pain and damage it may have caused while also fostering a compassionate space for growth and change. This journey invites men to deconstruct these limiting beliefs, allowing for the emergence of a more authentic, respectful and complete expression of masculinity.

"The ultimate measure of a man is not where he stands in moments of comfort and convenience, but where he stands at times of challenge and controversy." - Martin Luther King Jr.

Embarking on the quest for healthy masculinity means to set out on a transformative journey, one that calls for introspection, courage and a willingness to evolve. In Shadow Work, this quest is not merely a theoretical exploration but rather a deeply personal and transformative experience that holds the potential to reshape one's identity and interactions with the world.

Finding a way that we can identify as men again in a healthy way is at the heart of this journey. This quest is about being more open, inclusive and emotionally conscious. It's about redefining what it means to be a man in today's world, acknowledging the diverse ways in which masculinity can be expressed. By fostering an environment where men can be proud of their authentic selves, the journey towards healthy masculinity becomes a path of self-affirmation and growth.

Discovering healthy masculinity means unearthing our subconscious to explore and challenge the beliefs and norms they have internalized about what it means to be a man. Shadow Work becomes the go-to tool in this journey, guiding individuals to confront and embrace the aspects of themselves that may have been suppressed or neglected. This involves acknowledging both the strengths and the shadows within.

Healthy masculinity encourages men to be empathetic leaders, compassionate partners and emotionally intelligent individuals. It does not see vulnerability as a weakness but rather as a strength. By allowing oneself to feel and express a full range of emotions, men can forge deeper connections with themselves and others.

This quest is also about dismantling the harmful aspects of our unconscious patterns. It's about unlearning behaviors and attitudes that stifle growth and contribute to discord. Through Shadow Work, individuals can examine these internal structures, understand their origins and actively work towards cultivating a more balanced and authentic expression of self.

The journey towards healthy masculinity is about redefining strength, not as dominance over others, but as the courage to be genuine, respectful and kind. It's about recognizing the value in collaboration and the power in showing care.

In undertaking this quest, men are not only working towards their own personal growth but also contributing to a societal shift towards more inclusive and equitable understandings of gender. The quest for healthy masculinity is, therefore, not just a personal journey but a collective one, with the potential to bring about lasting change in individuals and communities alike.

> *"Strength lies in differences, not in similarities."*
> *- Stephen R. Covey*

Embrace Emotional Expression

Begin by allowing yourself to fully experience and express your emotions. Acknowledge that emotions are a natural part of the human experience and do not signify weakness. Practice verbalizing your feelings in safe spaces and cultivate a habit of introspection through journaling.

Challenge Traditional Norms

Take time to reflect on the societal expectations and norms related to masculinity that you've internalized. Question whether these align with your authentic self and consciously choose to let go of beliefs that are limiting or harmful.

Celebrate Diversity

Acknowledge and appreciate the diverse expressions of masculinity around you. Understand that there is no one-size-fits-all approach to being a man.

Cultivate Empathy

Actively work towards understanding and sharing the feelings of others. This can be done through active listening, practicing compassion and engaging in activities that promote connection and community.

Foster Vulnerability

Embrace vulnerability as a strength. Whether it's in relationships or personal growth, allowing yourself to be open and vulnerable can lead to profound connections and experiences.

Engage in Self-Reflection

Regularly practice Shadow Work to delve into your subconscious and explore the aspects of your personality and beliefs that need attention and transformation.

Pursue Balanced Relationships

Strive to establish relationships that are based on mutual respect, equality and open communication. Recognize the value of giving and receiving support.

Prioritize Self-Care

Pay attention to your physical, emotional and mental well-being. Engage in activities that nourish your body and soul, such as exercise, meditation and pursuing hobbies.

Encourage Others

Be a positive influence in your community by encouraging other men to explore and embrace healthy masculinity. Share your journey and insights in supportive environments.

Continuous Growth

Acknowledge that the journey towards healthy masculinity is ongoing. Be open to learning, evolving and adapting your understanding of yourself and masculinity as a whole.

Be Gentle with Yourself

Not everything you try might work out perfectly at first. Being patient and forgiving towards yourself will make your healing journey so much easier.

By integrating these practical steps into one's daily life, the quest for healthy masculinity becomes an attainable and fulfilling journey. Through Shadow Work, individuals are empowered to not only explore their shadows but also to illuminate their paths towards authenticity and growth. These steps are designed to create a ripple effect, fostering an environment where your masculinity is celebrated and nurtured. By actively engaging in this transformative journey, individuals contribute to a societal shift that honors masculinity, fostering a world that is enriched, balanced and harmonious.

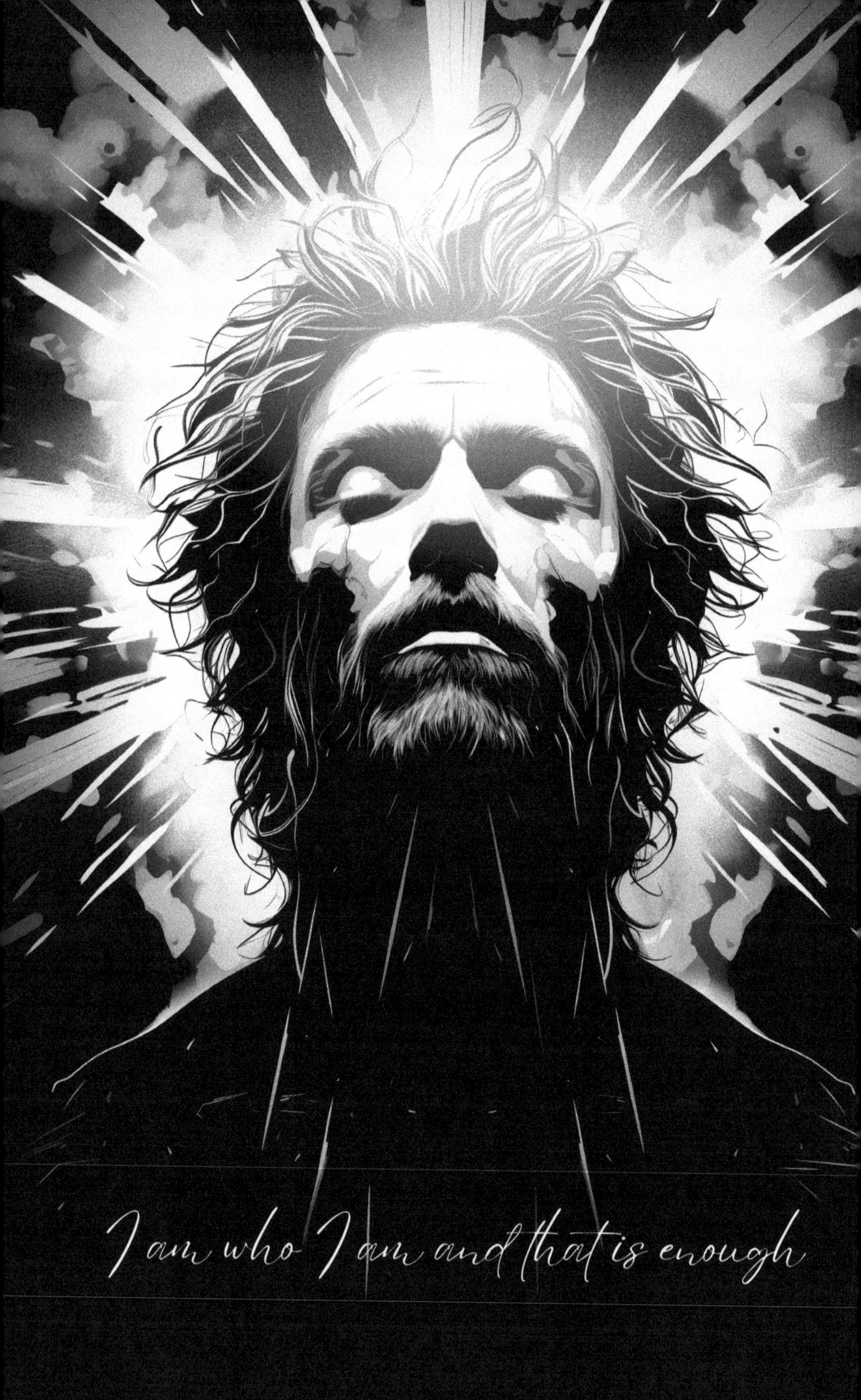

I am who I am and that is enough

CHAPTER THREE

Unmasking Emotional Armor

Understanding Your Defense Mechanism

"The walls we build around us to keep out the sadness also keep out the joy." - Jim Rohn

In the quiet sanctuary of solitude, have you ever found yourself peeling away layers, akin to a knight disrobing his armor after an arduous battle? Each piece falls with a clank, revealing a person beneath who is worlds apart from the warrior facade. This chapter invites you on a journey to explore and understand the emotional armor we men so often don – a protective suit that guards us from vulnerability yet distances us from our authentic selves and meaningful connections.

Imagine, if you will, a bustling metropolis. Amidst the concrete jungles and skyscrapers, every man is an island, armored in stoicism. We've been subtly conditioned to believe that emotions are akin to Achilles' heel – a fatal flaw that could crumble our very being. The 'man up' culture has been silently passed down generations, whispering in our ears that tears are a sign of weakness and that expressing feelings is a no-go zone.

So, we construct walls. Brick by metaphorical brick, we build fortresses around our hearts. These walls are laden with fears of rejection, ridicule and isolation. In trying to fit into the mold of the quintessential 'tough guy', we often find ourselves donning masks – be it the jester who laughs off pain or the stoic guardian who remains unfazed amidst pain.

Yet, herein lies the paradox: In our quest for connection and belonging, our emotional armor often becomes the very barrier that keeps us isolated. Picture a relationship, tender like a sapling yearning to grow. It requires the nurturing waters of vulnerability and the sunlight of authenticity. If we're armored, we're akin to a raincoat-clad gardener wondering why the sapling won't thrive. Our armor prevents the nurturing waters from reaching the roots.

"Your task is not to seek for love, but merely to seek and find all the barriers within yourself that you have built against it." - Rumi

Step 1: Acknowledge the Armor

Our emotional armor has been our silent companion, shielding us through life's tumultuous storms. It was our sanctuary during confrontations and our solace in solitude. The first step is to acknowledge this armor without judgment. It has served its purpose, protected us when we needed it the most and in many ways, allowed us to navigate through challenging situations. Take a moment to thank it for its service, recognizing its role in your life's journey.

Step 2: Identify the Layers

With acknowledgment comes understanding. This step requires introspection and self-reflection. Dive deep into your memories and experiences. When was the first time you felt the need to shield your emotions? Recall instances that led to the creation of this emotional armor. Was it a critical parent whose approval seemed unattainable, a playground bully who made vulnerability seem dangerous or a heartbreak that left scars? Identifying these layers is crucial, for it provides context and clarity to the walls we've built.

Step 3: Embrace Vulnerability

Vulnerability is often misconstrued as weakness, but in reality, it is courage in its purest form. It's the audacity to show up without any guarantees. To be vulnerable is to be authentically yourself, to embrace your emotions and experiences wholeheartedly. Start with small steps - share a fear or a dream with a close friend, express love unabashedly or allow yourself to feel pain without immediately seeking escape. This step is about dismantling the belief that vulnerability is a liability.

Step 4: Cultivate Emotional Agility

Emotional agility is the ability to navigate your emotions with precision and adaptability. Instead of resorting to the generic "I'm fine," explore the nuances of your emotional landscape. Are you feeling overwhelmed, elated, anxious or content? By giving voice to your emotions, you allow yourself to experience them fully and, in the process, gain insights into your own emotional complexity.

Step 5: Seek Support and Foster Connections

Unmasking doesn't mean leaving yourself defenseless. It's about discerning when to lower the drawbridge and let others in. Sometimes, the bravest thing you can do is to seek support, be it through friends, family or professional avenues. Forge connections that are nurturing and allow for emotional growth. Surround yourself with people who encourage authenticity and celebrate vulnerability.

Embarking on this journey of unmasking is like stepping into a realm of boundless possibilities. It is a liberating pilgrimage from the confining armor to the expansive freedom of authenticity. The journey might be challenging, fraught with moments of self-doubt and fear, but the rewards are immeasurable.

In essence, unmasking our emotional armor is a voyage home. It's a rediscovery of the language of our hearts, a reacquaintance with our authentic selves. It's about cultivating the courage to live unarmored, open and authentic. So, dear reader, let us embark on this transformative odyssey together. Let us break free from our self-imposed fortresses and step into a world that is rich with connection, authenticity and unmasked joy and laughter. This journey is not just about dismantling walls; it's about building bridges to a fuller, more authentic life.

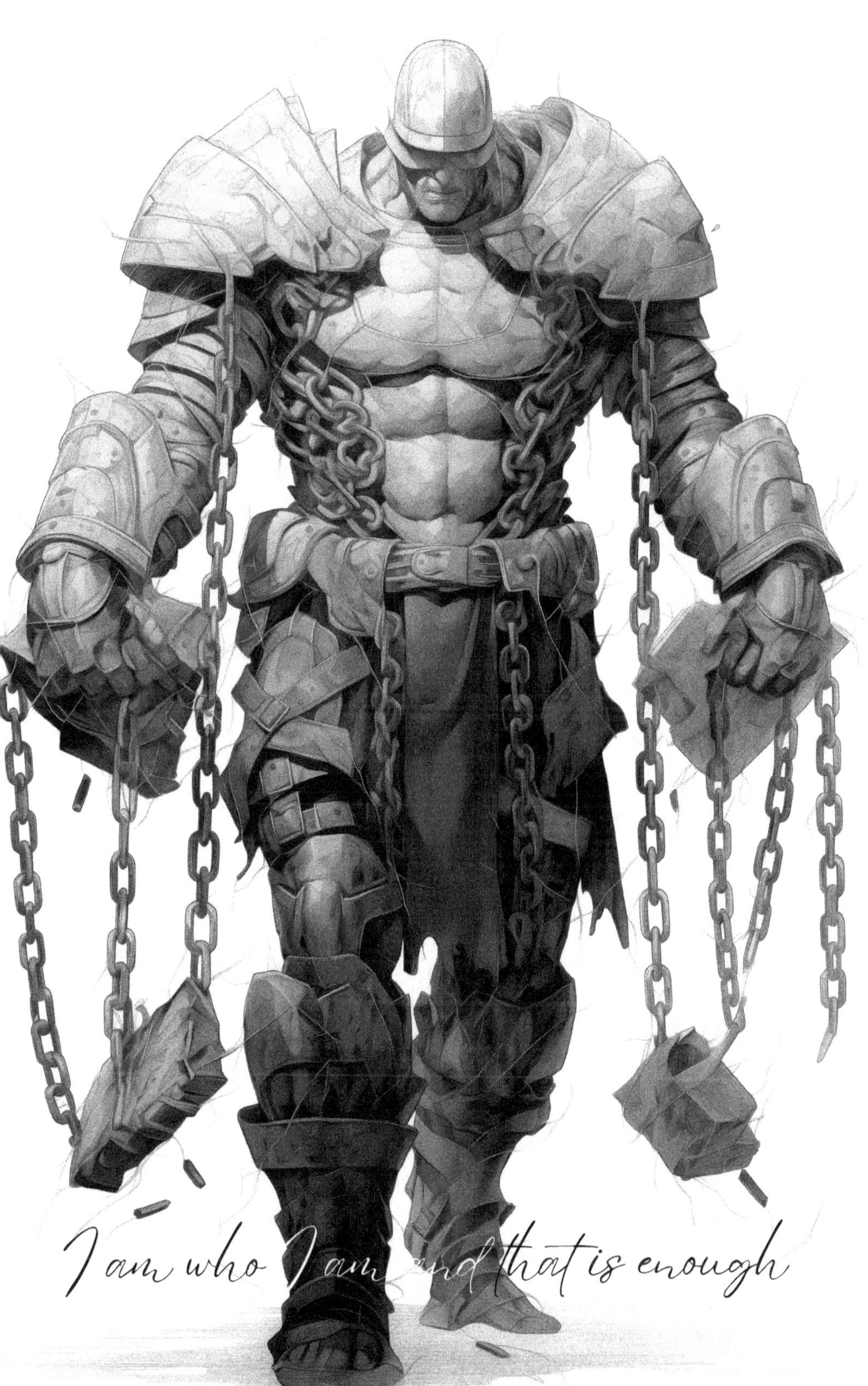

I am who I am and that is enough

CHAPTER FOUR

Emotions: Decoding Your Soul's Language

"Feelings or emotions are the universal language and are to be honored. They are the authentic expression of who you are at your deepest place." – Judith Wright

LOVE – WE ARE ONE

JOY – I'M TRULY ALIVE

SADNESS – I MISS A CONNECTION

ANGER – THIS ISN'T OKAY!

JEALOUSY – I DESIRE THAT TOO

FEAR – THIS ISN'T FOR ME

GUILT – I AIM HIGHER

SHAME – I EXPECT MORE OF MYSELF

Identify an Emotion: *Reflect on your recent feelings and identify the emotion that stands out the most to you.*

Decode the Emotion: *Considering that every emotion conveys a message, does this perspective alter how you relate to the emotion you've identified? If so, in what ways?*

Introduction: Deciphering the Heart's Code

Have you ever felt an emotion so intensely that words seemed inadequate? Perhaps it was a surge of pride from an unexpected compliment or a gut feeling warning you of something amiss. These moments can be seen as the heart voicing its distinct dialect—a language raw and potent, transcending any dictionary. This is your inner self's method of dialogue with you.

Why Emotions Are the Heart's Language

Visualize a child learning to talk. They start with sounds, progress to words and eventually form sentences. Our emotions evolve in a similar manner. Each emotion—joy, sadness, anger or satisfaction—is a character in the heart's language. As a child's vocabulary expands with experience, so does our emotional depth.

Favored Emotions & Unwelcome Visitors

We all have preferences, right? Preferred tastes, film categories, and certainly, emotions. We chase after joy, love and excitement as if they're the chart-toppers of our life's soundtrack. Then, there are emotions we'd rather skip—grief, discomfort, or envy. However, in the heart's language, every emotion is vital. Selectively embracing emotions is akin to omitting words from a language and expecting to grasp the full narrative.

Emotions as Silent Partners: Understanding the Bond

Think about the relationships you cherish. If someone consistently sought your support and was met with indifference, the connection would inevitably suffer. Disregard leads to misunderstandings, and eventually, the relationship weakens.

This concept is similar to how we interact with our own emotions. Dismissing feelings of sadness or avoiding anger is like telling parts of yourself that they don't matter. When neglected, these emotions can transform into shadows, quietly yearning for acknowledgment.

Cultivating Steadfastness

The principle of steadfastness revolves around preserving mental composure and balance, particularly in challenging circumstances. Viewing emotions as a language, equanimity becomes our interpreter. It guides us to attentively hear our heart's diverse tones without prejudice.

Illuminating the Shadows through Emotional Exploration

Consider Shadow Work as a fervent exchange of letters between your conscious and subconscious minds. It's raw, dramatic, enlightening and occasionally heart-wrenching. By acknowledging and interpreting these emotional correspondences, you begin to dispel the shadows that might be hindering your progress.

Here's how to commence:

Acknowledge All Emotions: Don't silence or trivialize any emotion. Greet each one as a visitor in your sanctuary.

Pursue Understanding: When faced with a formidable emotion, instead of retreating, inquire, "Why have you appeared? What insight do you convey?"

React with Respect: Even the most agonizing emotions seek recognition and respect. Address them with the same regard you'd extend to a brother-in-arms.

"One must talk to oneself and for oneself. This produces a dialogue and out of that dialogue one makes up one's mind." - Jiddu Krishnamurti

Engaging with the secret messages your emotions have been sending is crucial. But what comes next? Truly understanding and growing from these emotions involves not just hearing them, but actively engaging in introspective conversations.

The Strength in Acceptance

When Sadness quietly says, "I miss them," it's not beckoning you into despair. Instead, it's a subtle pull at your core, a nudge to remember. Begin by recognizing its presence without judgment. Embrace it openly and you might find it eases, paving the way for clear thinking.

Building Resilience through Responses

Anger may erupt, shouting, "My boundaries were breached!" Rather than retaliating or suppressing it, see it as a warning signal. What limits were overstepped? How can you reinforce or better communicate them? Use this as a chance to learn and stand firm in your space.

Affirming Bonds with Positive Reinforcement

When Love gently murmurs, "Our spirits connect," it's more than a comforting sensation. It's urging you to value, nurture and strengthen the ties you have. Pause to express thanks or perform a gesture of kindness. Even small acts can have a powerful impact.

Reflection over Suppression

If Jealousy prods you, whispering, "I deserve that too!" don't dismiss it. It could be directing you towards a neglected dream or goal. Instead of feeling defeated, introspect. Why does this stir within you? What steps can you take to close the gap between your current situation and your aspirations?

Daily Warrior Dialogues

Cultivate the habit of engaging in regular internal dialogues. It's like reconnecting with a trusted friend. Sometimes, a brief check-in can unveil deep insights. Comprehend their roots, honor their messages and incorporate their wisdom into your journey.

"The body never lies." - Martha Graham

Join me on an intriguing expedition through the expansive terrain of your body. Ever felt those flutters in your stomach before a crucial moment? Or the quickened heartbeat when someone captivating is near? These aren't mere physiological responses or the effects of caffeine; our emotions often manifest themselves physically.

First, let's explore the body's intuitive center: the gut. Have you ever experienced a deep "I just know" feeling that later turned out to be spot on? Some refer to the gut as our 'second brain'. So, when you feel an emotional storm brewing in your stomach, take a moment to ponder. Could it be a trace of nervousness for the upcoming meeting?

Next, let's focus on the heart, the constant beat that defines our existence. Feeling anxious? It races, mirroring your inner unrest. On a peaceful day, it beats steadily, aligning with your tranquility. In deeply emotional moments, each heartbeat is laden with emotion.

Now, onto the shoulders — our quiet carriers of stress. Notice how they tighten during challenging situations? When that occurs, imagine letting go of a hefty weight, symbolically releasing past regrets. It's a direct path to feeling at ease.

Let's journey down to the feet, our instinctive indicators. They may tap spiritedly to an upbeat melody or signal upcoming anxiety. They serve as both our rhythm companions and our grounding connection to the world.

Lastly, observe the hands. These dynamic conveyors often reveal more than intended. Under pressure, they may clench, a remnant of our ancestral survival instincts. In such moments, gently open your hands, releasing built-up stress and welcoming tranquility.

In essence, our body is not just a set of automatic reactions. It's an orchestra of signals, all interwoven, echoing with emotions and experiences. Periodically, pause to tune in. From your head to your toes, heed the stories they tell. Consider chronicling these experiences, crafting your own emotional map. By paying attention to and comprehending our body's stories, we access a profound level of self-awareness.

Shadows Within: Confronting Fear & Anxiety

"Fear keeps us focused on the past or worried about the future. If we can acknowledge our fear, we can realize that right now we are okay."
– Thich Nhat Hanh

Envision this: you're traversing the labyrinthine streets of an enigmatic ancient city. At every turn, signposts named fear or anxiety, sometimes both, glare in neon and emit a disorienting haze. These signposts are like intrusive pop-up ads – dramatic, slightly irksome, yet somehow functional.

Long ago, our forefathers navigated through the wilderness. A rustle in the foliage? They'd instinctively bolt in the opposite direction. Today, substitute that rustling with a pile of unread emails and you have a contemporary parallel. Recognizing this allows us to acknowledge fear and anxiety, appreciating their protective intent.

Have you ever heard the tale of the man who mistook a rope for a snake in the darkness, only to realize his error come daylight? A common misunderstanding, indeed. Yet, it illustrates a point: our minds, preoccupied with past traumas and hypothetical scenarios, may perceive threats where none exist. Anxiety can be that deceptive director, transforming mundane ropes into cinematic serpents. However, not every fear is a mere echo of past experiences. Sometimes, it's your inner compass subtly indicating, "This route? It's not the right one for us." Distinguishing genuine warnings from echoes of the past is crucial.

Caught in a tempest of panic? Let's engage in a grounding exercise with a twist.

See: Observe the colors around you. How many shades can you distinguish?

Touch: Feel the textures near you. Are they soft, rough, cold, or warm?

Hear: Focus on ambient sounds. Can you discern the furthest and the closest one?

Smell: Take a deep breath. Can you identify a familiar scent?

Taste: Savor the lingering flavor in your mouth, be it from a meal, drink, or simply the freshness of the air.

This exercise acts as your mental anchor, momentarily silencing the chaotic reel and anchoring you firmly in the present moment.

As you navigate your emotional terrain, do you observe when fear and anxiety take the spotlight? Maybe it's a subtle thumping in your chest or an unexpected chill on your arm. By tuning into these signals, we gain privileged insight into our emotional symphony. The challenge lies in determining whether these feelings are directing the main performance or simply contributing a unique nuance.

In confronting fear and anxiety, we uncover concealed harmonies. Beyond their initial intensity, these emotions can deepen our personal symphony, contributing richness, resonance and narrative depth. Thus, as we move through life's rhythm, remember: each emotion, including fear and anxiety, has a role to play. Embrace it, learn from it and continue the dance.

Dancing with the Fire: Unveiling Hidden Anger

"Speak when you are angry - and you'll make the best speech you'll ever regret."
- Laurence J. Peter

Let's delve into the fiery tango of anger. Picture yourself at a grand masquerade ball and Anger strides in, donning a bold mask, feathers flaring. Some guests might furrow their brows, muttering, "Who let them in?" But what if we adjusted our perspective? Visualize anger not as an uninvited intruder, but as the one who fiercely upholds the house rules, ensuring everyone's reveling in the festivities. Anger takes center stage, igniting the dance floor, when someone oversteps or attempts to switch our cherished tune. Ready to take the lead?

Rewind to our forefathers, navigating rugged terrains without today's comforts. For them, anger was a steadfast sentinel, ever vigilant, signaling, "Hold on! That's not right!" Recognizing the origins of anger allows us to acknowledge it even in our most heated confrontations, nodding, "Thanks for standing guard!"

Anger, however, has a certain flair—it doesn't always roar. Sometimes it's the silent, brooding guest in the corner, the biting toast or the swift exit from a cumbersome conversation. It's versatile: one moment, it's the commanding presence of Irritation, the next, the enigmatic guise of Passive Aggression. Recognizing its many faces ensures a smoother and more exhilarating dance.

Beneath anger's fiery cloak often reside tender emotions, perhaps even unshed tears. Concealed are the disappointments, the thwarted ambitions and those nagging doubts. So, when anger erupts, consider extending it a steadying hand and inquire, "What's truly at play here?" Brace yourself for revelations.

Remember our discourse on the emotional arsenal? Anger, that zealous warrior, seeks recognition. Channel its vigor into a thoughtful journal entry, a candid talk with a confidant or maybe a liberating dance session in your den. The aim? To articulate it with poise, ensuring it doesn't sound any alarms.

Now, when anger seems poised to ignite the ballroom, it's time to ground ourselves! Picture it as the cool-down phase after an intense duel. Visualize anger evolving, transitioning from a blazing flamenco to a composed waltz, until it gracefully bows and blends into the assembly. You've mastered the moves, and with that mastery comes the power to alter the pace.

Often, anger merely wishes to establish some ground rules. It's signaling, "Hey, stake out your territory!" But it's not about isolating oneself; it's about ensuring harmonious coexistence on the dance floor.

Embarking on this tempestuous dance with anger, we learn, spin and occasionally, falter. But with a steady rhythm and unwavering resolve, we can transform it into the most thrilling dance of our existence. So, as we march forward, bear in mind: every emotion, including our dance partner Anger, possesses its distinctive rhythm. Let's embrace it, move confidently with it and above all, relish the celebration!

Echoes of Solitude: Embracing Sadness, Loss and Loneliness

"There is a sacredness in tears. They are not the mark of weakness, but of power. They are the messengers of overwhelming grief and unspeakable love." - Washington Irving

Navigating the tangled paths of sadness and loneliness can sometimes feel like trying to find your way through a room of funhouse mirrors—everything's a bit distorted, with each reflection pulling at your heartstrings in unexpected ways.

Our ancestors were a tight-knit group, sticking close together not just for the latest tales by the campfire but because being alone was, quite literally, a dangerous game. Fast-forward to today, and even with our smartphones practically glued to our hands, that ancient feeling of "Uh-oh, I'm alone!" still taps us on the shoulder now and then.

If sadness were a foggy day, then processing loss is like trying to find your way through a particularly thick, pea-soup kind of mist. The kind where everything's blurry, but there's also a kind of quiet resilience as you discover your inner compass.

But hang on a sec—before we dive too deep into the blues, let's tip our hats to solitude. Think of it as the rugged cabin of emotions, secluded among the tallest trees. It's where you can kick back with a cold one, all while catching up on your favorite series or getting lost in a book. It's alone time, but with a touch of rugged charm.

Here's the great thing about sadness, loneliness and those moments when you feel like you've misplaced your emotional map: They're like your personal GPS, signaling, "Hey, maybe it's time to call up that old buddy!" or "How about reliving some legendary memories?" They're not nagging; they're gently suggesting routes toward healing and brotherhood.

When these emotions start feeling like they've overstayed their welcome, imagine them as waves. Rather than getting caught in the undertow, stand your ground. Let each wave pass, knowing that every retreat carves out a bit more strength, wisdom, and, believe it or not, a sense of humor in your soul.

Life, with all its twists and turns, stitches together moments of sorrow, solitude, and loss, crafting a tapestry that's uniquely yours. Amid these threads, there's room to weave in vibrant stories of hope, camaraderie, and the next epic adventure.

"Shame corrodes the very part of us that believes we are capable of change." - Brené Brown

That slight discomfort you feel when you indulge in sweets and then recall your neglected fitness routine? That's Guilt, gently nudging you with a reminder of your wellness aspirations. It's not about fixating on the misstep, but rather a subtle push towards improvement for the next time.

Shame on the other hand questions your worth as a person. Guilt points out the step you faltered on, shame ponders whether you're even fit to dance at all. The distinction is clear: Guilt zeroes in on the action, while shame probes into identity. Yet, there's a certain magic – your interaction with Shame determines its sway over you. Rather than allowing it to judge your worth, become inquisitive. What triggers this profound resonance? By delving into its roots, you can turn this melancholic ballad into a melody of empowerment.

So, how do you navigate these emotions? First, identify that emotional stir. What's it communicating? Guilt or Shame? Then, probe deeper. What kindled it? Perhaps an old recollection or a recent incident? And this is where the excitement commences. Engage with these emotions. Extend a reassuring nod, a soothing touch.

The Garden of Growth: Insecurity and Self-Worth

"You yourself, as much as anybody in the entire universe, deserve your love and affection."
- Buddha

If you've ever tried gardening, even just potting a plant, you'll agree it's not just about the plants. It's about the soil, the sunshine, the care and sometimes, the sneaky weeds that pop up when you're not looking. Our inner world, dear reader, is not so different.

Picture this: Your mind as this sprawling garden. You've got your majestic trees – those are your big wins, your strengths. Then there are these brilliant blooms of joy and passion. But, hey, what's a garden without some drama? Enter the weeds of Insecurity and Lack of Self-Worth.

Insecurity is sneaky, always whispering, "Are you sure about that? Do they really like you?" But here's the plot twist: Insecurity, with its sneaky tendrils, isn't all bad. When acknowledged, it might just point out where you need a bit more sun or water, metaphorically speaking. Dive into its roots, ask, "What's eating you?" You might just find a pocket of your garden that's been thirsting for attention.

Then we have the bush of Lack of Self-Worth. A bit thorny, this one. It sits there, sometimes making you feel more hedgehog than man. But within, oh within, are the buds of your true value, waiting to bloom. Those prickles? They're just challenges, tests of resilience guarding the precious core of you. Nurture this bush, approach it with care, and remind yourself: I am worthy of every drop of sun and rain.

Gardening, like soul-searching, takes work. It demands patience, introspection, and yes, occasionally dealing with bugs and weeds. But that's the beauty of it. Every challenge, every weed, is just an invitation to grow, to adapt, to flourish even more radiantly.

A little tip from one gardener to another: When those weeds start to feel too wild, take a moment. Feel the sun on your face, appreciate the blooms you've cultivated, and the sturdy trees you've grown. You're not just a gardener; you're the heart of this verdant paradise."

Reflection on Emotions: *Which emotion(s) resonated with you the most when reading this chapter? Why?*

Behavioral Transformation: *Based on what you've learned from this chapter, what specific behaviors or habits do you feel inspired to change or adopt? How do you plan to implement these changes?*

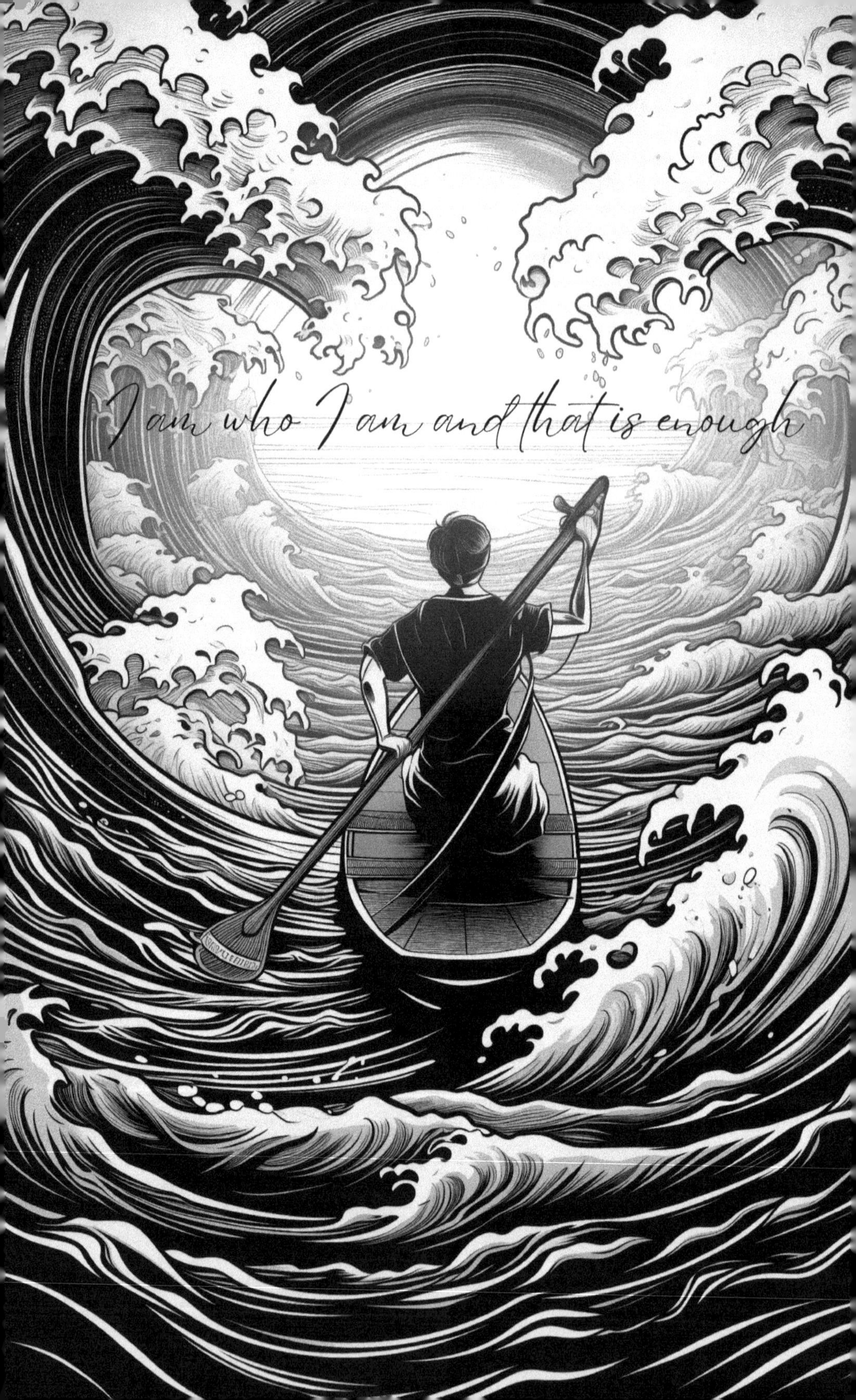
I am who I am and that is enough

CHAPTER FIVE

Trauma Healing Techniques That Work

*"The wound is the place where the
Light enters you."* — *Rumi*

Navigating the intricate maze of our personal wounds and emotions has brought us to this moment of reflection. Before delving further, it's essential to understand the trajectory of trauma healing, which largely falls into three defining stages.

Stage 1: Waking up to your Trauma - This is where most find themselves. A dawning realization, characterized by reading books, watching videos, or perhaps seeking therapeutic counsel. Yet, while there's abundant talking and thinking about the trauma, change remains elusive. The old patterns continue to resurface, playing out in a repetitive loop. It's not uncommon for many to linger here for years, often unknowingly.

Stage 2: Trauma Processing - The journey intensifies. Here, thinking gives way to doing. One starts delving deeper, confronting those haunting memories and emotions head-on. It's the emotional and somatic work that takes precedence. This stage is much like a rollercoaster – fleeting moments of triumph, followed by frustrating regressions. The teetering between past patterns and newfound awareness is palpable. Yet, with time and persistence, one begins to notice genuine shifts in behavior and personality.

Stage 3: Awakening - A stage where life is embraced in all its raw authenticity. Gone is the tumultuous rollercoaster, replaced by a profound resilience and equilibrium. There emerges a consistent confidence, a universal love and a profound connectedness to all around us, heralding our deep communion with the universe.

As we transition from our recent discoveries, we're primed to journey further into the realm of healing and reconstruction. The broken mirror of our past, marked by fragmented and sometimes distorted reflections, beckons for restoration. Yet, this journey isn't merely about mending; it's about evolving. Our goal is to reshape this mirror into a beacon of clarity, strength and wisdom.

Healing, in its essence, is both an art and a process. It beckons us to select the apt tools, foster the right mindset, and seize those defining moments of action. This chapter goes beyond sharing techniques. It's a heartfelt invitation to deeper self-awareness, illuminating not just who you were, but the boundless potential of who you can become.

So, with a mix of anticipation and curiosity, let's immerse ourselves in the practices that promise to guide our journey to healing.

Whispers from the Past: Engaging with Your Inner Child

"It's never too late to have a happy childhood."
- Tom Robbins

Ever had that moment, sitting around the dinner table at a family gathering, and you and your sibling dive into a "Remember when…" story, but it feels like you're talking about two different planets? I mean, same living room floor for building Lego castles, same cartoons giving you Saturday morning life lessons, same parents giving you the "Because I said so!" speech. Yet, your memories? As different as apples and oranges!

Picture it this way: two artists, same sunset, yet one paints with warm oranges and reds, and the other captures hues of purples and blues. You and your sibling? Both painting your childhood with your unique color palettes. Maybe your brother was the golden boy with the halo, while you sometimes felt like you had to pull off a magic trick just to be noticed. It's wild, right? How the same house can feel like a castle for one and maybe just a tiny bit like a dungeon for another. Every interaction, be it with parents, friends or the kind stranger at the candy store, gets stored differently in our heart's memory vault. And in that vast sea of childhood memories, each little version of us holds a personal diary of emotions and tales.

Close your eyes. Think summer, age seven. Feel the sun on your skin. What are you wearing? Sneakers or sandals? Are you happy, or are those tiny brows furrowed? Dive into that. Or maybe another age is calling out to you? Twelve? Fifteen? That embarrassing day in high school? Go where your heart pulls. Trust me; it knows its way around.

Once you're there, imagine you're sharing a giant cookie and just... talk. "Hey, how was school today?" or "What made you so upset at that birthday party?" Open up the lines, and you'd be amazed at the stories that tumble out. And hey, journal this. I promise, the patterns that emerge? Worth it.

Ever felt a weird flutter in your heart when someone forgot to call? Or that heavy lump in your throat when you entered a room full of strangers? These might just be the younger you tugging at your shirt, reminding you of moments they felt left behind or scared. These triggers? They're your roadmap. Dive in, explore, get curious. But remember, it's your journey. Your triggers, your landmarks. All unique.

But understanding is just the appetizer. The main course? Reparenting. Imagine if you could be the superhero for your younger self. Scoop them up, tell them they're seen, heard and so very loved. This is your shot. Through conscious self-reparenting, you're not just patching up old boo-boos, you're belting out a lullaby for those old scars, letting them know it's okay to heal.

Missed that bedtime story? No worries! Become the storyteller. Craved for a comforting voice? Be that voice. Be the parent, the friend, the mentor you needed. Lay down that new track of love and understanding.

Embracing your inner child is like rekindling a deep, soulful relationship from the past. Each interaction is a blend of rediscovery, tender moments and invaluable lessons. While the journey of reconnection can be lengthy, its rewards are profound and transformative. Consider this the very heart of trauma healing. Commit to this practice regularly, and watch as it becomes a guiding light on your path to healing and wholeness.

Childhood Safe Haven: Recall your childhood safe space. Describe its ambiance and how it made you feel secure.

Parental Traits: *Reflect on one positive and one negative trait you inherited from your parents. How do they influence you?*

Joyful Moments: *Remember a moment of pure childhood joy. What sparked that happiness?*

Childhood Fears: *Think of a fear you had as a child. How did you cope with it then?*

Lessons from Mistakes: *Recall a childhood mistake and the lesson it taught you.*

Message to Inner Child: *Write a short, comforting message that your inner child needs to hear today.*

Navigating the Minds Labyrinth: The Power of Cognitive Behavioral Therapy

"You can't stop the waves, but you can learn to surf." - Jon Kabat-Zinn

Are you ready to embark on a mind voyage? Close your eyes. Imagine a situation that left you anxious or upset. What were you thinking? How did your body react? Was your heart racing like a sprinter at the starting line? Were your thoughts a tangled web? Now, imagine if you could untangle that web, thread by thread and attain a sense of calm and control.

To practically use CBT in your life, start by identifying and writing down your negative thoughts in a journal. Next, challenge these thoughts by questioning their accuracy and considering alternative perspectives. For instance, ask yourself if there's evidence supporting your negative thought or if there's a more positive way to view the situation. Gradually, practice replacing negative thoughts with more balanced and constructive ones.

CBT is about recognizing those automatic negative thoughts and questioning, "Hey, is this really true?" or "Is there another way to see this?" It's like being both a detective, investigating your thoughts and a diplomat, negotiating with them.

Ever felt that sinking sensation when plans go awry? Or that flutter of panic at the thought of speaking up? These might be echoes of past experiences, shaping your present reactions. By decoding these echoes through CBT, you understand and gently reshape them. It's similar to learning a new language - the language of resilience and balance.

Transformation through CBT is not just about eliminating the negative. It's equally about cultivating the positive. Imagine being the captain of your own ship, navigating through storms with grace and emerging stronger. You're not just dispelling clouds; you're learning to dance in the rain.

Each session, each insight, is a step towards a more balanced and resilient you. While the journey can be challenging, its rewards are immense and deeply empowering. Commit to this practice and watch as it becomes a beacon guiding you through the labyrinth of your mind.

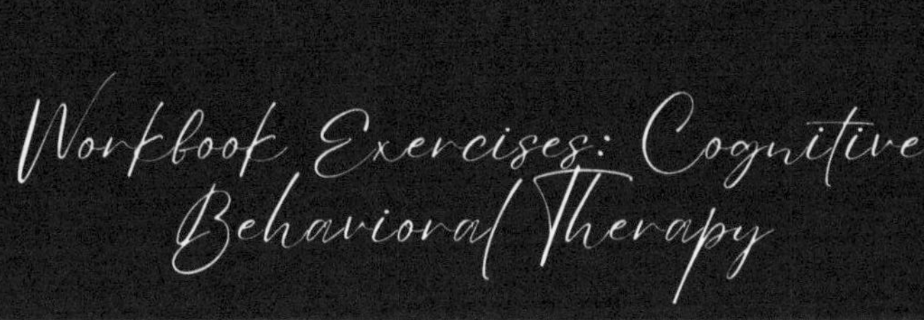

Mindful Moments: *Recall a situation that stirred strong emotions. What thoughts dominated your mind? How did your body react?*

Detective Work: *Can you identify any patterns or triggers that seem to set off a chain of negative thoughts? Describe them.*

Reality Check: *Think of a time when your initial negative thought was proven wrong. How did that make you feel? What did you learn?*

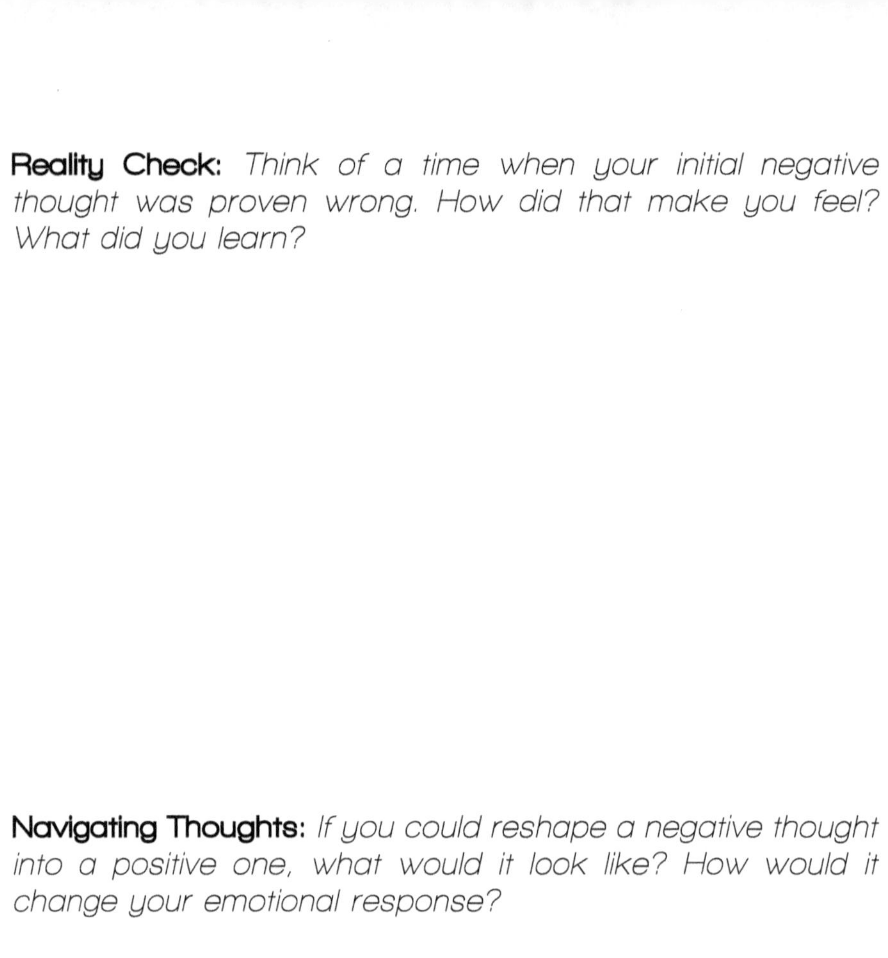

Navigating Thoughts: *If you could reshape a negative thought into a positive one, what would it look like? How would it change your emotional response?*

Captain's Log: *Write a letter to yourself from the perspective of a future you who has mastered CBT. What advice and encouragement would they offer?*

"Trauma in a family can resemble a relay race. Pain sprints from one generation to the next until someone breaks the cycle." - Kristin Jones

Ever felt a strange, inexplicable fear, or found yourself facing issues that seem far bigger than your personal experiences would warrant? Well, there's a chance these aren't just your traumas. They could be the whispers of generations before you, passed down like old family recipes or heirloom jewelry. This is the realm of generational trauma.

Generational trauma, sometimes known as ancestral or intergenerational trauma, refers to the transfer of trauma from one generation to the next. If your grandparents or great-grandparents endured significant traumas, the emotional fallout of those experiences can echo through the family tree, touching branches far and wide.

Science is still delving deep into this, but emerging research suggests our genes can carry memories of traumas experienced by our ancestors. When events are that emotionally charged, they can leave a mark on our DNA, subtly influencing our behaviors, beliefs and reactions.

Alright, time-traveler, now that we've dipped our toes into the pools of the past, how can we cleanse these waters for future generations? The first step is awareness. Recognizing that certain patterns or fears might not originate from our personal history can be liberating. It's like realizing you've been carrying a backpack filled with rocks that aren't even yours.

From there, shadow work becomes crucial. By diving deep into these ancestral patterns, we can start to heal not only ourselves but our lineage. It's like being the superhero your family lineage didn't know it needed.

A beautiful way to start is by charting your family history. Talk to elders, discover stories and find patterns. Journal about them. This doesn't mean you'll solve the puzzle overnight, but each piece you lay down lights the path for both past and future generations. So, grab that lantern, and let's illuminate those generational shadows together.

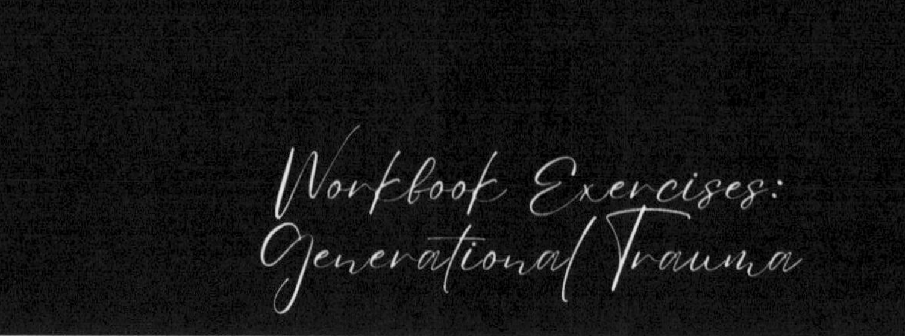

Ancestral Echoes: *Are there any recurring stories or patterns you've noticed in your family history?*

Emotional Inventory: *List down any fears, reactions, or behaviors you have that don't seem to connect directly to your personal experiences. Could they be remnants of generational trauma?*

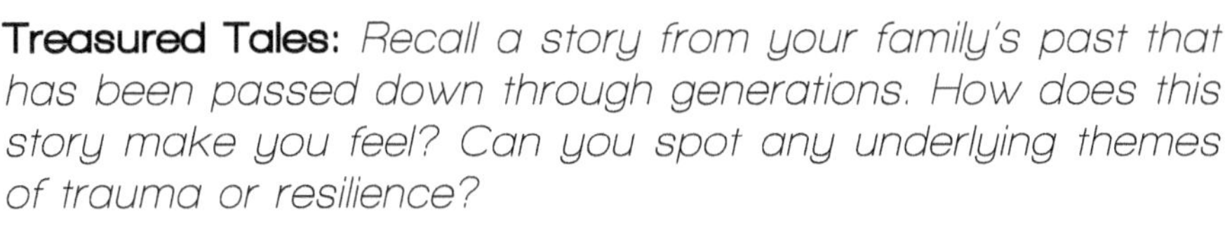

Treasured Tales: *Recall a story from your family's past that has been passed down through generations. How does this story make you feel? Can you spot any underlying themes of trauma or resilience?*

The Healing Hero: *If you were to imagine healing a specific trauma from your family's past, what would it look like? How would it change the narrative for future generations?*

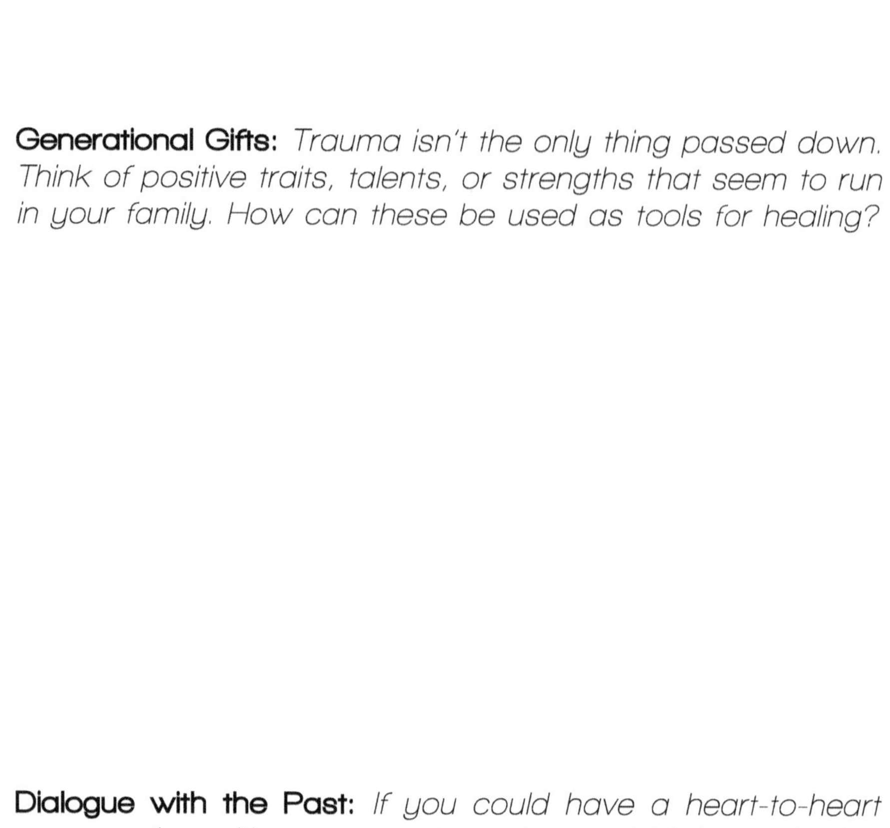

Generational Gifts: *Trauma isn't the only thing passed down. Think of positive traits, talents, or strengths that seem to run in your family. How can these be used as tools for healing?*

Dialogue with the Past: *If you could have a heart-to-heart conversation with any ancestor, who would it be and what would you ask or say?*

Dreams for the Future: *Envision a future where you've played a role in healing your family's generational trauma. What does it look like for your children, grandchildren, or even great-grandchildren?*

Reflection on Resonance: *Which technique(s) felt just right or spoke to you most deeply? Why?*

Mapping the Journey: *How do you envision incorporating your chosen technique(s) into your daily, weekly or monthly rhythm?*

I am who I am and that is enough

CHAPTER SIX

Doing Shadow Work Like a Pro

"The most terrifying thing is to accept oneself completely." - Carl Jung

Envision yourself as Sherlock Holmes, the famed detective donned in his signature deerstalker hat. Your shadow is like Dr. Moriarty, cleverly hidden, but revealing itself in unexpected moments. Just as Sherlock always catches Moriarty, we're going to do the same with our shadow.

Overreaction - The Emotional Flare-ups

Ever snapped at someone for a minor thing? Or maybe you've been on the receiving end of someone's inexplicable anger? This might be the shadow at play. Our overreactions are often the outcome of unresolved emotional trauma or suppressed emotions. So, next time you feel that surge of emotion, instead of brushing it off, grab your metaphorical magnifying glass and delve deeper.

Projection - The World's a Mirror

If you've ever thought, "Why is everyone else so _____?", that blank might be a piece of your shadow. Often, the qualities we dislike in others are the ones we don't accept in ourselves. That colleague who's "too bossy" or the neighbor who's "always showing off" could mirror the traits you've suppressed.

Repetitive Patterns

Ever wondered, "Why does this always happen to me?" Be it relationships, jobs or any recurring life situations — these patterns often have a shadowy root. They're the universe's way of pointing towards aspects we need to address.

Triggers and Defense Mechanisms

"Oh, I always avoid talking about that!" or "I usually make jokes when I feel uncomfortable." These are defense mechanisms that protect us from confronting our shadow. Any topic or situation that makes us uncomfortable or defensive might be holding a clue to our shadow. Embrace vulnerability. The next time you feel defensive, pause and ask yourself, "What am I protecting?"

Emotional Flare-ups: *Reflect on the last time you overreacted to a situation. Write down the specifics of what happened. What do you think might have been the deeper emotion or suppressed memory at play? How did you feel immediately after the event?*

Mirror, Mirror on the Wall: *List down three traits or behaviors you've recently observed in others that irked or bothered you. For each trait, write about a time you might have displayed that behavior or felt the urge to. What emotions arise as you reflect on this?*

Patterns in Play: *Think of a recurring event or pattern in your life. Describe it in detail. What emotions or thoughts do you associate with this repetitive cycle? If your shadow could speak through this pattern, what do you think it would say?*

Trigger Points & Shields: *Identify a topic or situation that you actively avoid or get defensive about. Dive into why it makes you uncomfortable. If you had to face this head-on, what's the worst and best thing that could happen?*

"The cave you fear to enter holds the treasure you seek." - Joseph Campbell

Alright, adventurers of the psyche, it's time to roll up our sleeves and get personal. Remember those whispers in your ear when you least expect them? That voice which seems to nudge you in unexpected ways? Yep, that's our shadow doing the talking. And guess what? It's high time we replied.

As with all the best conversations in life, start with an open heart. You wouldn't snap at a dear friend before they've even spoken, right? Your shadow, despite the somewhat ominous name, isn't some arch-villain. It's a piece of you. Treat it as you would an old friend you've lost touch with. Yes, there might be awkward pauses and hesitant starts, but oh, the stories it has to tell!

The shadow is born from our experiences. Every time we were told "big boys don't cry" or "good girls stay quiet", parts of us were pushed into the shadows. This suppression wasn't out of malice; often it was a protection mechanism, keeping our fragile selves from heartbreak, rejection, or shame. Recognize that your shadow's formation wasn't about being 'bad' or 'wrong'. It was simply coping.

This isn't an interrogation. No harsh lights and pressing demands. The shadow, after being hidden for so long, might be wary. After all, it's seen the sharp end of suppression and rejection. Approach it with gentleness, understanding and patience. It's not about prying open locked doors but waiting for them to be opened from the inside.

As you delve deeper, you'll find moments of revelation. Why you bristle at certain comments, why specific songs stir a whirlwind of emotions or why certain scents take you back decades. It's a journey of unraveling and understanding. And, every step of the way, you're not alone; you're in the best company—yourself.

Think of the countless moments in your day where your mind drifts off just a bit—while waiting for your coffee to brew, taking a brief walk, or even during those idle moments in a shower. These moments aren't reserved solely for grand revelations or epic soul-searching sessions. Instead, they offer a chance to weave an ongoing dialogue with your shadow into the very fabric of your day-to-day life. The magic truly lies in this integration into everyday experiences. By consistently inviting your shadow into these simple moments, you're making a conscious effort to bridge the gap between the conscious and unconscious realms of your psyche. The goal is to foster a continuous thread of communication, ensuring you're always tuned in and receptive to its insights, whether it's hinting at a forgotten memory or signaling an old wound.

Making this dialogue with your shadow an integral part of your daily life doesn't just lead to fleeting moments of insight—it paves the way for deep-seated transformation. The more you practice this, the more profound your understanding and bond with that once-hidden part of yourself becomes. It's not just about acknowledging the shadow but about truly merging with it, allowing its wisdom to shape your responses, choices, and overall outlook. This is where the biggest shifts happen. Not in isolated introspective sessions, but in the consistent, day-by-day merging of the shadow with the conscious self. The result? A more harmonized, authentic and enlightened version of you.

First Words: *If you could say one thing to your shadow right now, what would it be? And what might it reply?*

Listening Practice: *Spend a few quiet moments today simply listening, without judgment. What does your shadow wish you knew?*

Mastering Shadow Integration with Ken Wilber's 3-2-1 Method

"The shadow exists only as unsymbolized thoughts, feelings, sensations and behaviors. When they are all symbolized and integrated, the shadow 'disappears' and only the Self remains."
- Ken Wilber

Alright, here comes the magic trick for transforming those shadowy parts of you! You've delved into the depths, faced those daunting parts and now? Now it's time to integrate. And how do you do that? Meet the 3-2-1 Method by Ken Wilber. It's as easy as, well, 3-2-1!

The Third-Person Perspective (3)

Start by thinking of your shadow aspect as 'it'—like it's a character in a book or a movie. Describe it. What does it look like? Sound like? How does it behave? By seeing your shadow as an 'it', you create a bit of distance. This gives you a chance to observe without getting emotionally entangled.

For instance: Instead of "I am always so angry," consider "There's a part of me that carries this anger."

The Second-Person Perspective (2)

Now, let's get a little personal. Address this shadow aspect as 'you'. Engage with it in a dialogue. Ask questions. Why are you here? What do you want? By treating your shadow as a 'you', you start building a relationship with it.

Imagine saying: "Hey Anger, why did you flare up during that meeting today?"

The First-Person Perspective (1)

Finally, it's time to fully embrace and own this part of yourself. This is where you refer to your shadow as 'I'. Feel it. Understand it. Befriend it. When you fully integrate it, it's no longer something you fight against but a part of who you are. Think: "I understand why I felt that anger. It's a part of me, and I am learning from it."

Now, a gentle reminder: this dance with your shadow is delicate and it demands patience. This isn't a race. You don't need to leap from one perspective to the next in haste. In fact, consider staying in each stage for a day or so. Allow the insights to simmer, the revelations to marinate. Be tender with yourself, granting the kindness and time you deserve. Because true self-understanding isn't a sprint; it's a lifelong marathon.

Reflecting the Shadow: The Mirror Technique

"Everything that irritates us about others can lead us to an understanding of ourselves." - Carl Jung

Ever caught your reflection in a mirror and wondered, "Is that really how I look?" Now, let's turn that physical reflection into a deeper, psychological one. The Mirror Technique is about using the external world as a, well, mirror, to identify, acknowledge, and heal the shadow parts of ourselves.

Step 1: Identify Reflections

Think of instances where you had strong reactions to someone else's behavior, whether positive or negative. These reactions are often your unconscious mind pointing towards a trait you possess but might not be fully aware of.

Example: Feeling a strong dislike for a colleague's arrogant demeanor.

Step 2: Self-Reflection

Ask yourself why you felt so strongly about that behavior. What does it reveal about your own beliefs, values, or suppressed traits?

Question: "Why does his arrogance bother me so much? Do I secretly crave the confidence he displays? Or am I suppressing a similar trait in myself?"

Step 3: Own and Integrate

If you identify a suppressed trait, own it. This doesn't mean acting out but acknowledging its existence. Then, think of healthy ways to express or channel this trait.

Action: "I recognize I too have a confident side I've suppressed fearing it might come off as arrogance. I'll focus on expressing my opinions more assertively in meetings."

Step 4: Gratitude for the Mirror

Every person or situation that triggers a strong emotion in you is offering you a chance to introspect and grow. Express gratitude for these mirrors in your life.

Mental Note: "Thank you, colleague, for unconsciously helping me recognize and integrate a part of my shadow."

By constantly observing our reactions and what they reveal about us, the Mirror Technique offers a direct pathway to not only recognize our shadows but also to embrace and integrate them in a constructive manner.

Cultivating a Relationship with Your Shadow Work Journal

"A journal isn't just a collection of writings, but a stage on which the self performs." - Irvin D. Yalom

Imagine, for a moment, being in a relationship with someone who never judges you, never interrupts and is always there for you, day or night. Sounds ideal, doesn't it? Well, good news! You already have access to such a relationship: it's the one with your journal.

Your Journal, Your Confidant

When beginning Shadow Work, your journal becomes more than just a tool. It turns into a confidant, a therapist, a friend. It doesn't ridicule or scorn. Instead, it offers a safe space for you to untangle the threads of your thoughts, feelings and experiences. Remember, it's not about writing for an audience; it's about writing for you.

Creating a Ritual

A relationship needs care, and like any other, your relationship with your journal flourishes with consistency. Create a ritual around your journaling time. Maybe light a candle, play music you enjoy or sip your favorite tea. This isn't just about writing—it's about immersing yourself in the experience.

Dates, Doodles, and Dreams

Feel free to personalize your journal entries. Date them, doodle in the margins, or stick in photographs or mementos. It's your space, and there are no rules. Over time, you'll find that these personal touches not only make journaling more enjoyable but also help you track your growth and transformation.

Having Conversations

It might sound a tad unconventional, but consider having a two-way conversation with your journal. Pose a question about a particular shadow you're grappling with and let your intuitive self-answer. This method can often lead to insights and resolutions.

Embrace the Evolving Relationship

Your relationship with your journal will evolve and that's okay! There might be days when you pour pages of raw emotions and others where you jot down a line or two. Some days, you might skip journaling altogether. Whatever the flow, honor it. Trust in the journey.

Remembering Your Why

When in doubt or feeling uninspired, remind yourself why you began this journaling journey. Your 'why' is the compass that'll steer you back to the pages, to introspection and to healing.

In closing, your journal is more than just paper and ink. It's a way of mapping your soul's journey, detailing the love you feel, the challenges you master, the growth you experience and of course the triumphs that are truly meaningful to you. So, treat it with kindness and reverence, for it holds the stories of your deepest dives and greatest ascents. Through thick and thin, in shadows and light, your journal stands by your side, ever patient, ever ready to embrace all that you are.

Reflection on Resonance: *Which technique(s) or rituals felt just right or spoke to you most deeply? Why?*

Mapping the Journey: *How do you envision incorporating your chosen technique(s) or rituals into your daily, weekly or monthly rhythm?*

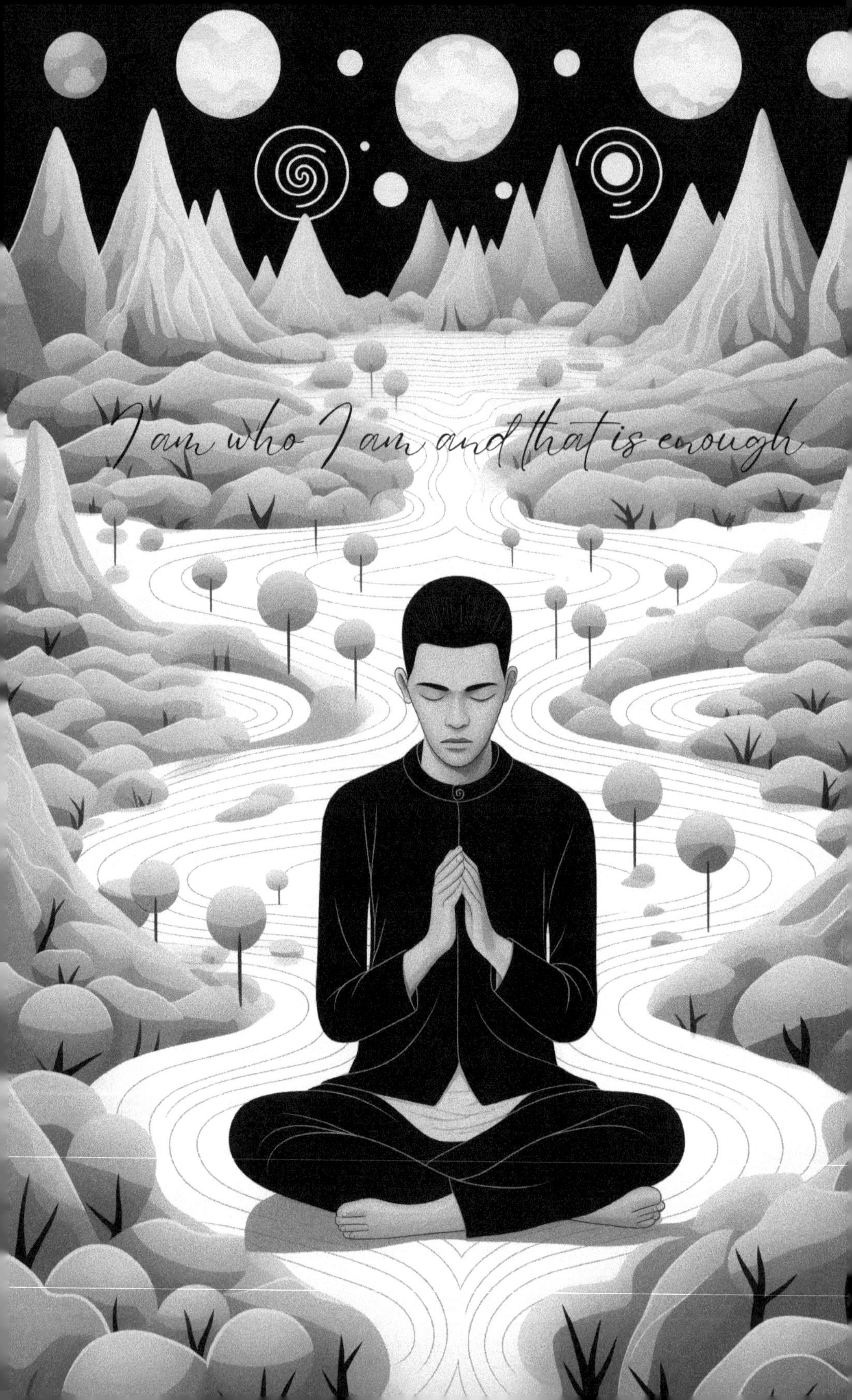
I am who I am and that is enough

PART II

Shadow Work Journaling Prompts

Reflect on a time when showing vulnerability felt challenging. Why was it difficult?

MASCULINE IDEALS

List societal expectations of masculinity that you feel pressured by. How do these align with your beliefs?

Describe a situation where you resolved conflict positively. What can you learn from this experience?

How do you define success? Does this definition align with your inner values?

List things you're grateful for and explore how focusing on them shifts your perspective.

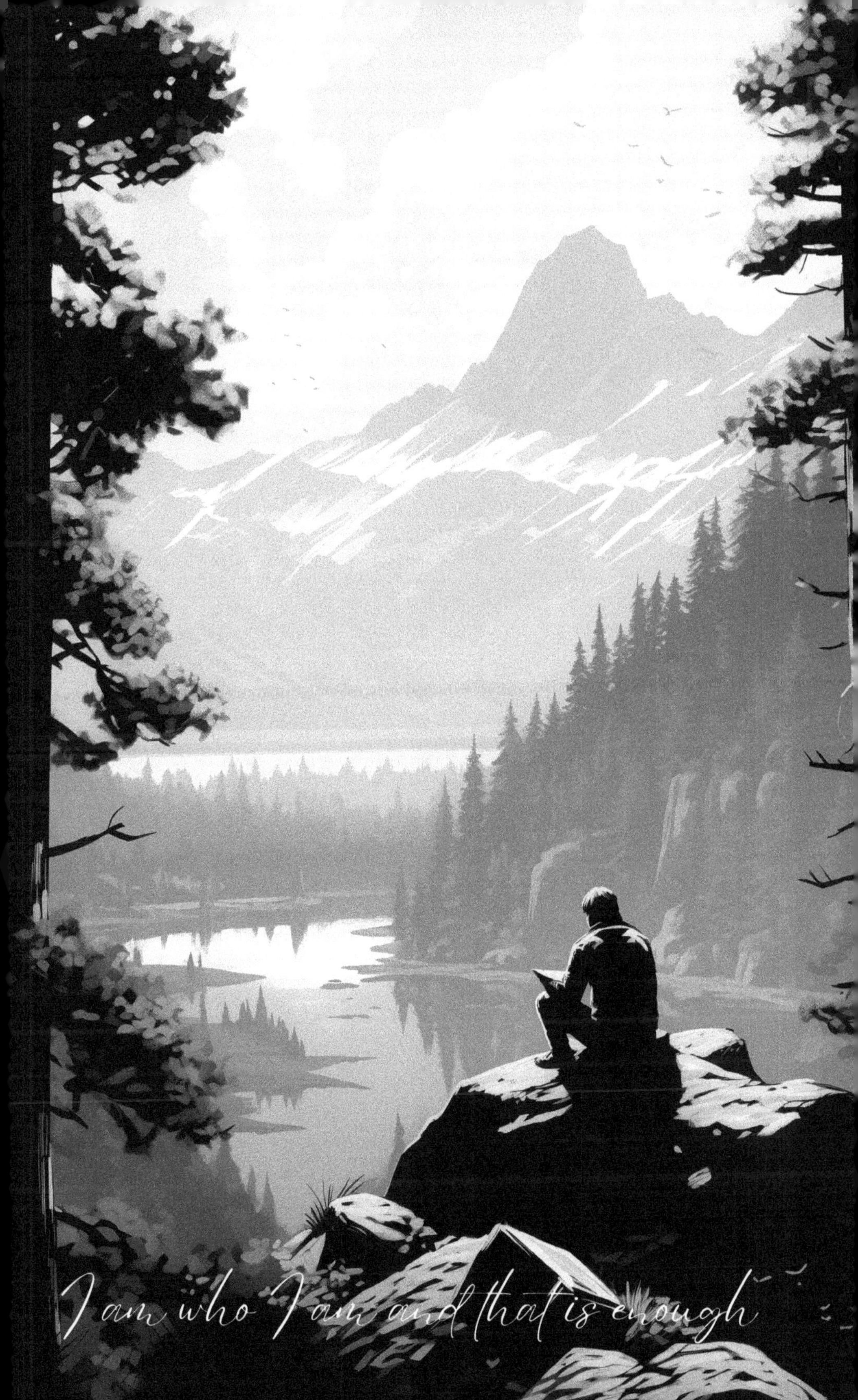
I am who I am and that is enough

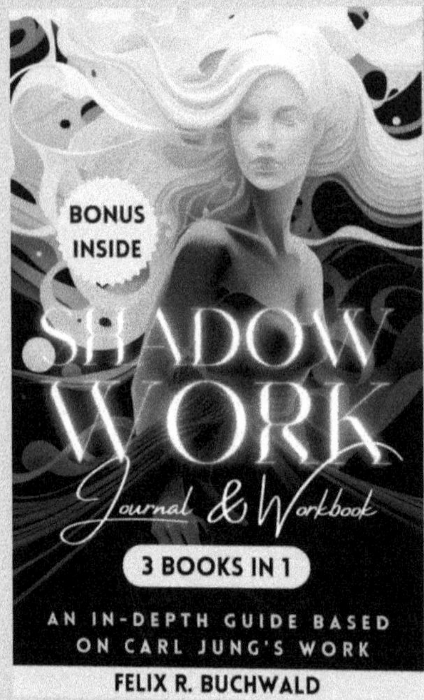

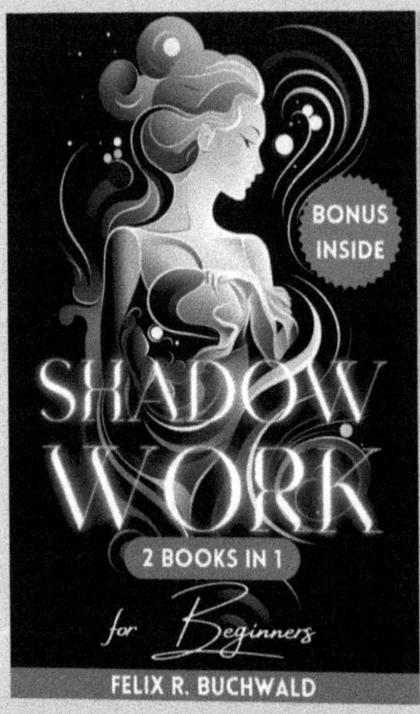

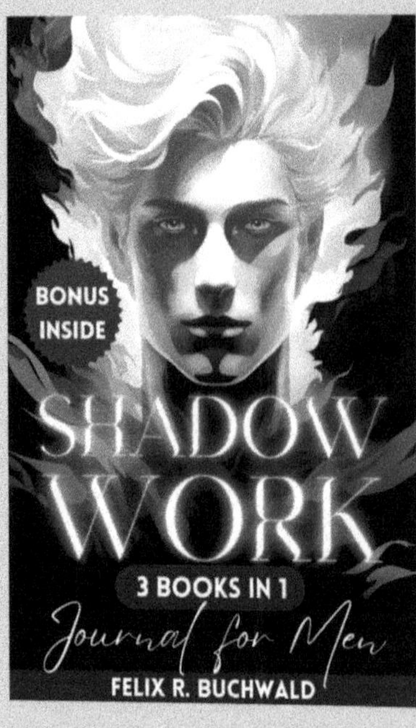

BOOKS BY
FELIX R. BUCHWALD

A HEARTFELT THANKS TO YOU!

Through shadow work, you heal not just yourself but also ripple healing to your family, community, and the world beyond.

Writing this book has been a transformative experience for me. I genuinely hope it brings you both joy and insight.

As a new self published author, your support means everything. Whether you leave a review on Amazon, share a glimpse of the book on social media, or choose to do both, it would make a world of difference. Thank you for being part of my journey!

QR Link to Amazon Review Page